Engaging patients
in healthcare

1

Engaging patients in healthcare

Angela Coulter

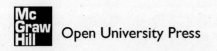 Open University Press

Open University Press
McGraw-Hill Education
McGraw-Hill House
Shoppenhangers Road
Maidenhead
Berkshire
England
SL6 2QL

email: enquiries@openup.co.uk
world wide web: www.openup.co.uk

and
Two Penn Plaza, New York, NY 10121-2289, USA

First published Open University Press 2011

A catalogue record of this book is available from the British Library

ISBN10: 0 335 24271 5 (pb)
ISBN13: 978 0 335 24271 9 (pb)
eISBN: 978 0 335 24272 6

Library of Congress Cataloging-in-Publication Data
CIP data has been applied for

Typeset by Aptara Inc., India
Printed in the UK by Ashford Colour Press, Gosport, Hampshire

Fictitous names of companies, products, people, characters and/or data that may be used herein (in case studies or in examples) are not intended to represent any real individual, company, product or event.

For Paddy

Contents

Preface

Improving responsiveness and securing greater patient and public engagement in healthcare is a central theme of health policy in many countries. This book gives an overview of the field, describing theories, concepts, evidence, policies and practical examples from the UK and abroad. It has been written for health professionals, students of medicine, nursing and allied health professions, social scientists, policy-makers, patients and interested laypeople. It is intended as a primer for all those who want to understand the various ways in which patient and public engagement could contribute to better health outcomes.

Patient engagement is a topic that arouses strong emotions. Some dismiss it as peripheral to the main business of healthcare, a fluffy notion that lacks the solid underpinning of scientific rigour on which medical care is supposedly built. Others are super-keen evangelists, preaching the gospel of patient engagement but taken aback by any suggestion that it should be subject to more dispassionate analysis. My starting point is one of strong commitment to the idea that patients and public should be more informed and involved, but as a researcher I believe the case for engagement ought to be rooted in an understanding of its impact on healthcare and health status.

Patient engagement is both as a means to an end, and an end in itself. It should be treated as an ethical imperative, but if it also leads to improved quality of care, more appropriate decisions, and better health outcomes, then it is much easier to persuade people that it is definitely worth while. To test this, we must look at the evidence and, as will become apparent, there are many theories and studies to be examined.

Readers in Scotland, Wales and Northern Ireland will notice a bias – most of the examples and policy references relate to England rather than the other UK nations. I hope they will forgive me for this – it would have been tedious to make constant references to the diversity of policies now in place in different parts of the UK and that was not the purpose of the book. Despite its anglocentrism, I hope the main arguments will be of interest and relevance to people outside England as well as those in it. The topic is a large one and the scope is broad, so I have included suggestions for further reading at the end of each chapter for those who wish to delve more deeply.

Acknowledgements

The book draws extensively on more than 25 years of studying patients' experience at the University of Oxford, the King's Fund, the Picker Institute and the Foundation for Informed Medical Decision Making. I owe a great debt of gratitude to my colleagues in each of these organizations, without whom none of this would have been possible.

The policy context

1

Overview

This chapter considers the reasons why successive UK governments in recent years have prioritized patient and public engagement. It outlines possible policy goals for individual and collective engagement and describes various roles that patients, families and communities can play. Finally, it introduces the topics covered in more detail in subsequent chapters.

The case for engagement

The UK has undergone considerable political, demographic and cultural change since the foundations of the NHS were laid down in 1948. New knowledge and new technologies have greatly expanded the potential of medical care to make a positive impact on people's lives and, more than 60 years on, the NHS continues to be a popular centrepiece of the British welfare state. But we are left with a significant problem – overdependence on technical solutions to health needs, the consequence of a failure to encourage self-reliance.

Modern medicine does indeed have a great deal more to offer than it did 60 years ago, but it cannot cure every ill, as some commercial and professional interests would have us believe. Over-treatment and mistreatment may now be greater threats to public health than under-treatment. Policy-makers are striving to shift the balance of care away from reliance on hospitals and complex technologies towards community-based care, but their efforts are meeting with little success. For years the dominant emphasis has been on professional knowledge, technical skills and expensive treatments. Dependence on the formal healthcare system has been encouraged, its limitations have been underplayed and an over-optimistic view of its therapeutic powers has been promoted. The central thesis of this book is that restoring a healthy equilibrium will require changes in the way professionals and services interact with patients. Instead of treating patients as passive recipients of care, they must be viewed as partners in the business of healing, players in the promotion of health, managers of healthcare resources, and experts on their own circumstances, needs, preferences and capabilities.

Challenging professional dominance

The history of public policy is a story of power battles between competing interests. In the first three decades of the NHS, the powerful combatants were professional bodies, trade unions and citizens (the electorate). Patients, as consumers of healthcare, did not really enter the fray until the 1970s when the first patient organizations began campaigning and the Community Health Councils (CHCs) were established. Initially, neither the CHCs nor the patient organizations wielded much power and for the most part their influence was restricted to specific campaigns (see Chapter 9). The decades since then have seen various attempts to give patients a stronger role in shaping health policy, led both by government and by external groups, with varying degrees of success.

The establishment of CHCs was an example of government trying to inject some grit into what was perceived as a professionally dominated and largely unresponsive service. This was the first of many policy initiatives aimed at encouraging greater responsiveness, several of which are described in more detail in later chapters. The problem that the government was trying to fix was described in graphic terms in *The NHS Plan,* which set out the Labour government's intentions for the service:

> The relationship between service and patient is too hierarchical and too paternalistic. It reflects the values of 1940s public services. Patients do not have their own health records or see correspondence about their own healthcare. The complaints system in the NHS is discredited. Patients have few rights of redress when things go wrong. The patient's voice does not sufficiently influence the provision of services. Local communities are poorly represented within NHS decision-making structures. Despite many local and national initiatives to alter the relationship between the NHS and the patient, the whole culture is more of the last century than of this. Giving patients new powers in the NHS is one of the keys to unlocking patient-centred services.
>
> (Secretary of State for Health 2000: 30)

Paternalism has been a defining characteristic of healthcare delivery in the UK for a long time (Coulter 2002). Doing things *to* people instead of *with* them can be profoundly disempowering. It encourages patients to believe that professionals have all the answers and that they themselves lack relevant knowledge and skills, and hence have no legitimate role to play in decisions about their healthcare. Paternalism breeds dependency, encourages passivity, and undermines people's capacity to look after themselves. It may appear benign, comfortable and reassuring, but it is a hazard to health. Exhorting people to choose healthy lifestyles carries little weight if they are treated as incompetent when they are ill.

The Labour government that came to power following the 1997 general election was determined to *'modernize'* the NHS. They hoped that empowered patients would act as a counterweight to professional dominance, strengthening the hands of managers charged with squeezing greater value out of the system. So the NHS Plan initiated proposals to amplify patients' voice and give them more choice in an attempt to create a subtle shift in the balance of power (see Chapter 2). The results of these efforts were mixed at best.

The Commonwealth Fund of New York organizes regular surveys in a selection of rich countries to monitor the performance of their health systems. In 2010 they monitored the quality of care in Australia, Canada, Germany, the Netherlands, New Zealand, the UK and the USA, ranking the countries according to six dimensions: quality of care, access, efficiency, equity, health outcomes and expenditure (Davis et al. 2010) (Table 1.1).

The UK performed reasonably well on most measures, but it was ranked next to last in respect of health outcomes such as preventable deaths, infant mortality and healthy life expectancy, and it was bottom of the pile for patient-centred care and patient engagement.

Promoting responsiveness

In 2010 a new Conservative-led coalition government was elected. They announced their intention to strengthen efforts to tackle both the problem of relatively poor clinical outcomes, and that of insufficient focus on patient engagement (Secretary of State for Health 2010). The new government's reasoning was similar to that of their predecessors:

> The NHS also scores relatively poorly on being responsive to the patients it serves. It lacks a genuinely patient-centred approach in which services are designed around individual needs, lifestyles and aspirations. Too often, patients are expected to fit around services, rather than services around patients. The NHS is admired for the equity in access to healthcare it achieves; but not for the consistency of excellence to which we aspire. Our intention is to secure excellence as well as equity.
> (Secretary of State for Health 2010: 8)

Retaining the previous government's focus on choice as a lever to drive up quality standards, the new government announced its intention to devolve responsibility for commissioning to local general practitioner-led consortia, putting clinicians 'in the driving seat'. Process targets were to be scrapped in favour of outcome indicators and all hospitals were to become Foundation Trusts, 'liberating' them from central control. To reinforce the message that the service was to be 'genuinely centred on patients and carers' they announced that shared decision-making between clinicians and patients should become the norm. Their White Paper trumpeted the slogan, 'no decision about me without me'.

Aside from politics, there are important reasons for thinking that engaging and empowering patients is the right way to go. Patients have been described

Table 1.1 Ranking of health systems in seven countries

	Australia	Canada	Germany	Netherlands	New Zealand	UK	USA
OVERALL RANKING	**3**	**6**	**4**	**1**	**5**	**2**	**7**
Effective care	2	7	6	3	5	1	4
Safe care	6	5	3	1	4	2	7
Coordinated care	4	5	7	2	1	3	6
Patient-centred care	2	5	3	6	1	7	4
Overall quality of care	**4**	**7**	**5**	**2**	**1**	**3**	**6**
Cost-related problem	6	3.5	3.5	2	5	1	7
Timeliness of care	6	7	2	1	3	4	5
Overall access	**6.5**	**5**	**3**	**1**	**4**	**2**	**6.5**
Efficiency	2	6	5	3	4	1	7
Equity	4	5	3	1	6	2	7
Long, healthy productive lives	1	2	3	4	5	6	7
Health expenditure per capita, 2007	**$3,357**	**$3,895**	**$3,588**	**$3,837***	**$2,454**	**$2,992**	**$7,290**

Note: *Estimate. Expenditures shown in $US PPP (purchasing power parity)

Source: Calculated by The Commonwealth Fund based on 2007 International Health Policy Survey; 2008 International Health Policy Survey of Sicker Adults; 2009 International Health Policy Survey of Primary Care Physicians; Commonwealth Fund Commission on a High Performance Health System National Scorecard; and Organization for Economic Cooperation and Development *OECD Health Data 2009* (Paris, OECD, Nov 2009). Reproduced from Davis et al. (2010) with permission from the Commonwealth Fund

as the greatest untapped resource in healthcare, suggesting that the quality and efficiency of healthcare could be improved if there was greater emphasis on helping them make better decisions (Kemper and Mettler 2002). This conviction was backed up by a body of research evidence suggesting that encouraging patients to play a more active role in their healthcare can increase their knowledge and enable them to manage their health better (Coulter and Ellins 2007). Thus there was good reason to hope that active engagement of individuals, families, voluntary organizations and communities could improve the effectiveness and productivity of the health service.

Policy goals

So what might be the goals of a more patient-centred approach to health policy? This question is surprisingly absent from many of the writings about patient and public involvement. The moral case for encouraging greater involvement is usually assumed, with most of the effort focused on mechanisms rather than objectives. Of course it is very important to learn how to do it better, but unless goals are clarified and outcomes articulated we are left with no means of measuring progress.

It is helpful to consider the needs of patients and public (citizens) separately. What we want as individual patients and how we articulate these needs can be distinguished from our collective aspirations as citizens or members of the public (Coulter 2005). As citizens we may be concerned about abstract notions of what constitutes a 'good' service, for example: affordability; efficiency and value for money; universality, equity and fairness; safety and quality; health protection and disease prevention. As patients, we do not lose our citizen concerns at the door of the GP surgery or the hospital, but we naturally prioritize our own interactions with the system, especially with the health professionals who deliver our care. So in general, patients care more about the quality of their everyday interactions with health professionals than about how the service is organized, whereas citizens often care passionately about perceived threats to the NHS and the values it is seen as representing. Involving citizens means opening up the debate about the pattern and nature of service provision, while engaging patients involves tackling the clinical agenda and, where necessary, changing the culture of care. Individual engagement includes concepts such as personalization and choice, whereas collective engagement is concerned with strengthening the public voice, by encouraging democratic accountability and ensuring that the health system is responsive to people's needs and preferences. The contrasting goals that might follow from a focus on individual or collective engagement are shown in Table 1.2.

Monitoring progress towards these policy goals is easier said than done. Unfortunately health services research does not employ a standard set of outcome measures that are easy to summarize. However, in two overviews of the effectiveness of patient-focused interventions, we found that outcome

Table 1.2 High level policy goals

Individual engagement – focus on patients	Collective engagement – focus on citizens
To improve the quality of care and patients' experience	To increase public understanding of health issues
To ensure appropriate and effective treatment and care	To promote health and reduce inequalities
To help people live independently for as long as possible	To increase research-based knowledge and encourage innovation
To promote safety and reduce harm	To promote efficient use of resources
To reduce complaints and litigation	To strengthen accountability
To improve health outcomes	To build social capital

measures could generally be categorized into four main groups: impact on knowledge; on experience; on service utilization and costs; and on health behaviour and health status (Table 1.3) (Coulter and Ellins 2006; Picker Institute Europe 2010).

The patient's role

Since the publication of the NHS Plan, patient and public involvement (PPI) has become part of the everyday rhetoric in the NHS. Everyone knows that they have a responsibility to encourage it, but few have deconstructed it, critically assessing its specific relevance and application to their particular service. As a result, efforts have often been restricted to consulting local people about planned service developments, or securing lay membership on a raft of committees and policy-making bodies. These activities are valuable in themselves, but they hardly scratch the service of the fundamental change that would be required if the ambitious goals outlined above were to be realized. In particular, they do little to challenge the prevailing clinical culture that affects the everyday experience of patients. If patients are to be active participants in their care, health professionals must be willing and able to support their efforts.

People can play a distinct role in promoting the health of themselves, their families and their communities by:

- understanding the causes of disease and the factors that influence health
- diagnosing and treating minor conditions
- knowing when to seek advice and professional help
- choosing appropriate health providers
- selecting appropriate treatments
- monitoring symptoms and treatment effects

- being aware of safety issues and preventing errors
- coping with the effects of chronic illness and managing care
- adopting healthy behaviours to prevent occurrence or recurrence of disease
- ensuring that healthcare resources are used appropriately and efficiently
- participating in clinical and health services research
- articulating their views in debates about healthcare priorities
- helping to plan, govern and evaluate health services
- working collectively to tackle the causes of ill health.

Table 1.3 Outcome measures

Patients' knowledge	For example: • Knowledge of condition and long-term complications • Self-care knowledge • Knowledge of treatment options and likely outcomes • Comprehension of information • Recall of information
Patients' experience	For example: • Patient satisfaction • Doctor–patient communication • Confidence to manage health problems • Patient involvement • Self-care activities • Social support
Service utilization and costs	For example: • Hospital admissions • Emergency admissions • Length of hospital stay • GP visits • Cost-effectiveness • Cost to patients • Days lost from work/school
Health behaviour and health status	For example: • Quality of life • Psychological well-being • Treatment adherence • Symptom control • Functional ability • Clinical indicators of disease severity • Lifestyle and health-related behaviour

Source: Reproduced from Coulter and Ellins (2007) with permission from the BMJ Publishing Group Ltd

Of course, most people do manage minor illness without recourse to professional help and many play an active role in several of the other tasks listed above. But, as will become clear in subsequent chapters, the system and culture of care does little to strengthen their ability to perform these roles, sometimes actively undermining it. It is important to consider the extent to which people might be willing to take on more responsibility for their health. Could this be seen as placing an additional burden on people when they are ill and feeling vulnerable? The evidence is reviewed in more detail later in the book, but in general it shows that there is a demand for a new kind of relationship, albeit with variations depending on the people involved, the setting and context. Could there be a downside to responding to the desire for greater participation? Is there a risk that shifting the balance will undermine people's trust and confidence in the healthcare system?

Trust

Trust is fundamental in healthcare, both because it is a key component of the therapeutic relationship, and because it is intrinsic to the principles of social solidarity and fairness that underpin confidence in public healthcare systems. However, trust is not the same as blind faith. Nowadays, few people are willing to place unconditional trust in clinicians, organizations and systems (Calnan and Rowe 2008). Instead trust has to be earned. Clinicians earn patients' trust by demonstrating their competence and technical skills, by communicating clearly and effectively, and by showing empathy. Managers earn it by ensuring that healthcare facilities are accessible, clean, safe and efficiently run. The NHS earns it by providing free care to all those who need it as promptly as possible. Mutual trust is also important – many patients expect clinicians to trust them, as well as the other way around. This means trusting patients to act as effective decision-makers, care managers, and co-producers of health and supporting them in these roles. It seems unlikely that championing open and honest communications and giving people the opportunity to influence decisions would undermine trust. On the contrary, it may prove to be essential for maintaining it.

The rest of this book is structured around eight policy priorities or objectives (see Figure 1.1). Each chapter looks at the rationale for engaging patients or citizens in the particular task, outlining what is known about their willingness to get more actively engaged and the likely effects if they are encouraged to do so. Ways in which the various tasks can be strengthened are explored, clarifying concepts and comparing different approaches. The final chapter reviews what we have learnt and considers likely future developments.

A note on terminology

It is easy to stumble into semantic minefields when writing about patient engagement. For a start, both words 'patient' and 'engagement' are fraught with

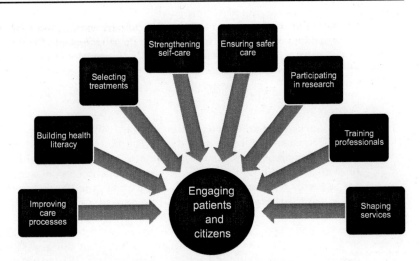

Figure 1.1 Patients' and citizens' contribution to policy priorities

difficulty. Use of the term 'patient' is highly controversial in some quarters, mainly because of its implied association with two other nouns, 'patience' and 'suffering'. In fact the *Shorter Oxford English Dictionary* gives a neutral definition: 'A person receiving or registered to receive medical treatment' that describes almost all of us in the UK accurately (if we are registered with a general practice). This dictionary states that an old meaning of the term, 'a person who suffers patiently', is now considered obsolete.

Some people have suggested that we should cease using the term 'patient' altogether because it implies that recipients of healthcare have inferior status, but none of the suggested alternatives are really an improvement (Herxheimer and Goodare 1999; Neuberger 1999). 'Client' is the term given to people who seek help from social workers, accountants, lawyers and other professionals, but this word can also mean 'a person who is under the protection of another; a dependent, a hanger on'. Both 'consumer' and 'customer' suggest a financial relationship involving purchasing or using a commodity, implying that public health services operate like commercial markets. As purchasers of services, consumers have some power over providers who have a vested interest in responding to their needs (Coulter 2002). For this reason some people prefer the term 'consumer' and it has been adopted by various groups, but others reject it on the grounds that consumerism is an individualistic concept that fails to capture the collectivist essence of health systems. People working in mental healthcare and some groups representing people with long-term conditions often use the term 'service user' in acknowledgement of the fact that these groups often have multiple needs that go beyond medical services, but it is a clumsy word that implies a relationship with an inanimate object instead of an active partnership. It also carries connotations of drug misuse and can therefore be easily misunderstood. Instead of adopting a different word, it might be better to adapt the definition. I have suggested changing it to 'co-producer of health; autonomous partner in treating, managing and preventing disease' (Coulter 2004).

In the meantime I have chosen to use 'patient' throughout this text except when one of the other words seemed a better fit.

'Engagement' is an even more difficult word to define and the *Shorter Oxford English Dictionary* is not very helpful here. The term has numerous meanings, including some quite contradictory ones; for example, 'bind by a promise of marriage', 'enter into combat', 'provide occupation for', and 'come into contact with or fit into a corresponding part so as to prevent or transmit movement'. The most relevant definitions for our purposes are 'attract and hold fast a person's attention'; 'enter upon or occupy oneself in an activity, interest, and so on'. Thus the act of engagement can be both transitive and intransitive, active or passive, done by or done to. It can also be used to describe the motivations and actions of all parties, patients and providers, healthcare organizations and communities. But these definitions are broad and non-specific. What is needed is a definition that applies to engagement in healthcare. The Center for Advancing Health in the USA has suggested the following: 'actions that individuals must take to obtain the greatest benefit from the healthcare services available to them' (Center for Advancing Health 2010: 7). The trouble with this is that it excludes actions taken by health professionals or healthcare organizations and it assumes that individuals must act alone. I prefer to see engagement as a set of reciprocal tasks, as follows: 'working together to promote and support active patient and public involvement in health and healthcare and to strengthen their influence on healthcare decisions, at both the individual and the collective level'.

The terms used to describe people who work in health services can also be confusing. When I have used the word 'clinician', I mean to include all people with a clinical role; that is, doctors, nurses and allied health professionals; while 'health professional' has been used in an even broader sense, to include all the aforementioned plus healthcare managers.

Summary

Since the latter part of the twentieth century, UK governments have made various attempts to improve the responsiveness of the NHS to patients' needs and preferences. Despite these efforts, healthcare in the UK appears less patient-centred than those in several other rich countries. An engagement strategy should take account of the varying requirements of patients and citizens, adopting clearly specified objectives and monitoring progress carefully. The maintenance of trust in the health system and between patients and clinicians will be important.

References

Calnan, M. and Rowe, R. (2008) *Trust Matters in Health Care*. Maidenhead: Open University Press.

Center for Advancing Health (2010) *Snapshot of People's Engagement in their Health Care*. Washington, DC: CFAH.

Coulter, A. (2002) *The Autonomous Patient: Ending Paternalism in Medical Care*. London: Nuffield Trust.

Coulter, A. (2004) When I'm 64: Health choices, *Health Expectations*, 7(2): 95–97.

Coulter, A. (2005) What do patients and the public want from primary care?, *British Medical Journal*, 331(7526): 1199–1201.

Coulter, A. and Ellins, J. (2006) *Patient-focused Interventions: A Review of the Evidence*. London: The Health Foundation.

Coulter, A. and Ellins, J. (2007) Effectiveness of strategies for informing, educating, and involving patients, *British Medical Journal*, 335(7609): 24–27.

Davis, K., Schoen, C. and Stremikis, K. (2010) *Mirror, Mirror on the Wall: How the Performance of the US Health Care System Compares Internationally*. New York: Commonwealth Fund.

Herxheimer, A. and Goodare, H. (1999) Who are you, and who are we? Looking through some key words, *Health Expectations*, 2(1): 3–6.

Kemper, D. W. and Mettler, M. (2002) *Information Therapy: Prescribed Information as a Reimbursable Medical Service*. Boise, ID: Healthwise Inc.

Neuberger, J. (1999) Let's do away with 'patients', *British Medical Journal*, 318: 1756–1758.

Picker Institute Europe (2010) *Invest in Engagement*. Oxford: Picker Institute Europe, Department of Health.

Secretary of State for Health (2000) *The NHS Plan: A Plan for Investment, A Plan for Reform*. London: The Stationery Office.

Secretary of State for Health (2010) *Equity and Excellence: Liberating the NHS*. (Cmd. 7881). London: The Stationery Office.

2 | Improving care processes

Overview

This chapter looks at ways in which patients can be involved in improving care processes and ensuring that healthcare delivery responds to their needs and preferences. After considering various policy levers, including those that aim to promote 'voice' and 'choice', we examine what is meant by patient-centred care and how it can be measured. Various quality improvement mechanisms, including patient feedback, financial and organizational incentives, provider choice and patients' charters are assessed, and examples of approaches that involve patients directly in quality initiatives are described.

Policy levers

How to deliver high-quality healthcare in the most efficient manner possible is the question that obsesses policy-makers in the twenty-first century. While there may be disagreement on how to achieve this goal, most analysts and policy-makers agree that healthcare delivery should be:

- **Clinically effective:** focusing on treatment outcomes, including survival rates, symptoms, complications, patient-reported outcomes, and indicators of well-being and independence.
- **Safe**: avoiding harm, looking after people in clean, safe environments, and reporting any medical errors or adverse events.
- **Equitable:** ensuring that healthcare is available to all according to need and avoiding financial barriers that prevent access to necessary care.
- **Efficient:** paying attention to value for money, avoidance of unnecessary interventions, and careful stewardship of limited resources.
- **Responsive:** providing personalized, patient-centred care, delivered with compassion, dignity and respect; measuring, analysing and improving patients' experience and satisfaction.

Healthcare systems in many developed countries are in an almost constant state of change as policy-makers search for ways to match the supply of healthcare to the demand for it. They struggle with the requirement to balance competing priorities and contain costs in the face of ageing populations and increasing expectations (Figure 2.1).

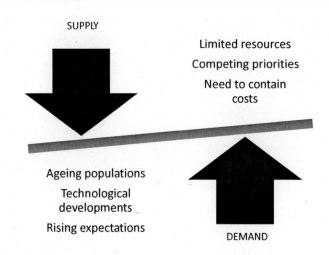

SUPPLY

Limited resources
Competing priorities
Need to contain
costs

Ageing populations
Technological
developments
Rising expectations

DEMAND

Figure 2.1 Balancing supply and demand

Most efforts to reform health systems are attempts to find the holy grail of higher quality at lower cost. Six main levers for change have underpinned most initiatives in the field of healthcare reform in recent years (Dixon and Alakeson 2010; Le Grand 1999):

- **Trust:** Professionals and managers are trusted to know what is best for patients and it is assumed that they will deliver high-quality healthcare with minimal interference from government or regulators.
- **Command and control:** The government directs the process by issuing directives or guidance or by setting performance targets for healthcare providers, with rewards and penalties to encourage compliance.
- **Financial incentives:** Commissioners are given fixed budgets to purchase healthcare services for their local populations, governments or regulators determine the prices and payment mechanisms for specific clinical interventions or care processes, pay-for-performance is offered to incentivize improvements, and financial penalties are levied for failure to achieve minimum standards.
- **Competition and choice:** Patients are encouraged to choose from a range of competing providers, which may be publicly or privately owned and run, and money follows the patients, which should incentivize providers to raise standards in order to attract patients.
- **Regulation:** Organizational and economic regulators, usually independent of government, set the rules of engagement and accredit providers against a core set of standards, using performance measurement to assess compliance.
- **Voice:** Patients are encouraged to express their views (compliments and complaints) through direct feedback or via advocates or elected representatives in the hope that this will encourage providers to improve standards.

Each of these approaches has influenced health and social policy thinking in the UK and all have been tried, often simultaneously, sometimes accompanied by robust political debate about their relative merits and likely effects. Efforts to improve responsiveness to patients' needs and wishes have deployed each of the levers to varying effect. Much of this effort has been focused on improving patients' experience of care and ensuring that services are patient-centred.

Patient-centred care

The term 'patient-centred care' is widely used but there is often confusion about what it means (Mead and Bower 2000). Ensuring that care delivery is responsive to patients' physical, emotional and social needs, that interactions with staff are informative, empathetic and empowering, and that patients' values and preferences are taken into account is the essence of patient-centred care. This is considered important not just because people want it, but also because patients' experiences can influence the effectiveness of treatment and health outcomes. Sometimes referred to as person-centred care, patient-focused care, or personalized care, the aim is to ensure that healthcare is 'respectful of and responsive to individual patient preferences, needs, and values, and ensuring that patient values guide all clinical decisions' (Institute of Medicine 2001). Berwick has suggested an improvement on this definition:

> The experience (to the extent the informed, individual patient desires it) of transparency, individualization, recognition, respect, dignity, and choice in all matters, without exception, related to one's person, circumstances, and relationships in health care.
>
> (Berwick 2009: w.560)

In recent years there has been a distinct shift away from paternalistic ways of thinking about the patients' role, in which the need to treat people with dignity, respect and compassion was recognized but they were not viewed as active players in their own care. Nowadays professionals are encouraged to treat patients as co-producers of health and as autonomous partners in treating managing and preventing disease. This concept has been summarized in a useful catch phrase: 'Nothing about me without me' (Delbanco et al. 2001: 144).

Scientific advances have transformed healthcare since the mid-twentieth century and the influence of evidence-based medicine, a concept first described in the early 1990s, has fuelled huge advances in knowledge about what works and what does not. However, these developments have come at a cost, namely the tendency of biomedical science, with its focus on 'hard' science, to marginalize and undervalue the 'softer' notions of caring, compassion and respectful delivery of healthcare. Planetree, a US-based organization specializing in improving patients' experience, has called on staff and organizations to refocus on improving interactions and relationships with patients and their families. They underline the enormity of the task and the need to radically change organizational culture: 'The change in human interactions that is the core of a patient-centred approach requires a monumental shift in attitudes' (Brady and Frampton 2009: 288). The key issue is how to embrace the best of evidence-based medicine while regaining a focus on patients' individual and emotional needs.

Patients' priorities

Several key themes emerge whenever patients are asked about their priorities. What most people want is the security of knowing that health services will be there when they need them, that their views and preferences will be taken account of by health professionals, that they will be given the help they need to help themselves, that they can access reliable information about their condition and the treatment options, and that they will not have to worry about the financial consequences of being ill. They also want health professionals to empathize by showing that they understand what it feels like to experience illness and undergo treatment, to anticipate their needs for information and support, and to treat them in a kindly and dignified manner.

Interpersonal skills are at the heart of a patient-centred approach. A review of the literature on patients' priorities for general practice care found that the most important factor was 'humaneness', which ranked highest in 86 per cent of studies that included this aspect. This was followed by 'competence/accuracy' (64 per cent), 'patients' involvement in decisions' (63 per cent), and 'time for care' (60 per cent) (Wensing et al. 1998). The nature of patients' relationships with their primary care doctors is particularly important, especially for older people who tend to place greater value on continuity of care as they become more frail.

Much of the relevant research has focused on identifying and measuring the various features that comprise the concept of patient-centred care. A number of bodies, including the Institute of Medicine, the Institute of Family-centred Care, the International Alliance of Patients' Organizations, Planetree and the Picker Institute, have deconstructed the notion of patient-centredness into various components, with a broad consensus on the key features:

- Good communications, emotional support and empathy
- Provision of reliable and comprehensible information
- Involvement in decisions about treatment and care
- Education and support for self-care
- Personalization of services, coordination and continuity
- Attention to physical comfort and pain relief
- Attention to privacy, confidentiality and dignity
- Involvement of family and friends
- Fast access to appropriate help and advice when needed.

These attributes are important, not just because people prefer to be treated by clinicians who are good listeners and good at informing, advising and educating them, but also because it is hoped that this type of care may contribute to better health outcomes. There are indications that patient-centred care may indeed improve outcomes. For example, studies have found that patients whose treatment is deemed patient-centred are more likely to trust their clinicians (Keating et al. 2002), more likely to adhere to treatment recommendations (Haynes et al. 2008), and less likely to die following a major event such as acute myocardial infarction (Meterko et al. 2008).

Monitoring the quality of care

The question of how well the NHS is performing is a constant focus of attention among politicians, the media, those who work in the service and those who use it. Statistics are gathered routinely on almost every aspect of care to monitor performance, including numbers of consultations and numbers of patients treated, diagnoses, treatments and procedures, workforce numbers, waiting times, hospital admissions and lengths of stay, mortality rates and cause of death, prevalence of health-related behaviours and risk factors. Numerous reports are published and regularly scrutinized by politicians, regulators, researchers, journalists, and members of the public interested in assessing NHS performance to determine whether quality is improving or getting worse.

Of particular interest is what patients have to say about their experience of using the service. In the UK and many other countries, relevant information can be gleaned from national patient surveys that are regularly carried out by governments, regulators and other bodies. For example, an overview of the results from 26 national patient surveys, including responses from more than one and a half million NHS patients in England gathered between 2002 and 2007, drew the following conclusions (Richards and Coulter 2007):

- **Communications:** Confidence and trust in health professionals was high on the whole and most patients gave positive reports about their interactions with NHS staff. However, hospital patients said they sometimes found it difficult to find a doctor or nurse willing or able to talk to them about their fears and concerns.
- **Information:** Most respondents said they usually received clear, comprehensible answers to their questions, but staff sometimes failed to anticipate their information needs and often did not provide adequate information about care processes, treatments and likely side-effects. Only a minority of patients referred to specialists had been given copies of their referral letters.
- **Involvement:** When asked whether they had been involved in decisions about their care as much as they wanted to be, a third of primary care patients and half of hospital patients said they had not been sufficiently involved.

- **Support for self-care:** Many hospital patients said neither they nor their family members were given sufficient advice on how to care for themselves when they went home, and many of those with long-term conditions would have liked more information and education for self-care.
- **Coordination:** About a third of hospital patients said they were sometimes given conflicting information by staff, and many of those with long-term conditions or mental health problems said they had not been involved in drawing up their care plans.
- **Physical comfort:** Having to sleep in mixed-sex wards or sharing bathrooms and toilets with members of the opposite sex, unappetizing hospital food, and noise at night-time were continuing problems noted by many hospital patients.
- **Privacy and dignity:** While most patients said they were treated with dignity and respect by staff, some complained of insufficient privacy when discussing their condition and treatment.
- **Family and friends:** Less than half of inpatients said that, on leaving hospital, their family or someone else close to them was given all the information they needed to help them recover.

Many of these problems had persisted throughout the five-year period under study, while a few showed slight improvement. Despite the problems, most patients gave positive assessments of their care overall. In general the survey results painted a picture of a service that was slowly improving but was still some way from achieving the goal of being truly patient-centred. Facilities and staff were not always as patient-friendly as they could be and opportunities to inform, support and engage patients as active participants in their own care and treatment were frequently missed.

Substandard care

Only about 2 per cent of patients report receiving poor care in NHS hospitals, but a minority of elderly people have received very substandard care. In 2009 the Patients Association published a report describing some examples of 'dreadful, neglectful, demeaning, painful and sometimes downright cruel treatment' received by elderly patients at the hands of NHS staff (Patients Association 2009: 3). Public concern about poor standards was heightened when shocking reports emerged from an inquiry into deaths at two hospitals in central England (The Mid Staffordshire NHS Foundation Trust Inquiry 2010). Family members gave heart-rending accounts of neglect of the needs of their elderly relatives and uncaring attitudes among staff.

Complaints about failure to provide prompt personal care were highlighted in both these reports:

There were a number of times I was shocked at the lack of dignity and compassion shown to her. She told me of one time that she had awoken in the night, dreadfully thirsty and unable to reach her drink. She pressed her buzzer for assistance. When the nurse arrived he said 'What do you mean by waking me at this time of night? What do you want? When I visited Ann … sometimes I found her lying in her own faeces. She would plead with them to change her, but the answer was always firm: 'We will get to you when we have time'. She didn't like disturbing the nursing staff, but she was totally compos mentis and she hated the indignity of it. One time the smell of urine from a neighbouring bed on the ward became almost overwhelming.

(Patients Association 2009: 32)

In the next room you could hear the buzzers sounding. After about 20 minutes you could hear the men shouting for the nurse, 'Nurse, nurse', and it just went on and on. And then very often it would be two people calling at the same time and then you would hear them crying, like shouting 'Nurse' louder, and then you would hear them just crying, just sobbing, they would just sob and you just presumed that they had had to wet the bed. And then after they would sob, they seemed to then shout again for the nurse and then it would go quiet…

(The Mid Staffordshire NHS Foundation Trust Inquiry 2010: 53)

Failure to help patients eat their meals in hospital was another common complaint:

There would be sweets or fruit or drinks on a table out of his reach. This is a common thing in hospital, that the person who brings the food doesn't put it within arm's length and make sure they are propped up enough to eat it. If you are lying down, you can't reach it or eat it.

(The Mid Staffordshire NHS Foundation Trust Inquiry 2010: 85)

Patients and their families are usually understanding about the pressures faced by staff, but when things go wrong it often seems to be because patients' and families' needs are not given sufficient priority:

At no time during my father's stay on the ward did we feel there was anyone who cared for patients enough and who took responsibility for ensuring they got the attention they needed. We often overheard staff complaining about how long they had been on duty and how much they missed working at another nearby hospital. Although staff complained to us about being overstretched we found many times it was difficult getting entry to the ward during visiting times. Had it been because staff were busy we would have understood, but looking into the ward we saw staff talking in groups at a desk. They did not respond to our request for entry until you called them via a mobile phone.

(Patients Association 2009: 11)

As I have said, from the simplest thing to the most important, keeping him out of pain was a priority. It had got to be; it was to us but it wasn't to them. It didn't matter if he had been lying there in hours of pain, as long as… In other words, on Ward 10 the patients revolved round the staff. If it was inconvenient for staff, it wasn't done. People could be calling for a bedpan or help to get to the toilet: yes, I will be back in a minute. Off they go and they weren't back in a minute. They had no intention of doing it, until people were just left to do it where they were. There was no dignity. There was no care. It was just totally dreadful... the nurses never spoke. They didn't know how to behave socially, I don't think.

(The Mid Staffordshire NHS Foundation Trust Inquiry 2010: 109–10)

International comparisons

Despite these horror stories, the NHS does tend to perform fairly well in international comparisons of the quality of care, with 86 per cent of UK citizens rating it 'good' or 'very good', compared to an average across European Union countries of 70 per cent (Spence 2010). NHS patients enjoy more equitable access to healthcare at lower cost than in most other rich countries and the primary care system is relatively strong (Schoen et al. 2009; Schoen et al. 2010). However, where it falls down in comparison to other countries is in the extent to which patients receive support from health professionals to play an active role in their own care (Coulter 2006). NHS culture appears more paternalistic than in many other developed countries health systems.

In response to evidence of slow and ultimately disappointing progress towards greater responsiveness on the part of all public services, not just health, in 2009 the British government stepped up its efforts to incentivize a more person-centred approach. Financial incentives were introduced in an attempt to make providers take the issue more seriously, regulators and commissioners were urged to take a tougher line, and citizens were encouraged to vote with their feet by exercising their right to choose alternative providers. The government returned to the task of promoting awareness of patients' rights and the focus on systematically monitoring the experience of service users, with regular feedback to providers, was stepped up.

Obtaining and using patient feedback

Obtaining systematic feedback from patients is seen as a key element in monitoring and improving the quality of healthcare. Feedback can be obtained using quantitative or qualitative methods (Table 2.1). It can be gathered during or after an episode of care. It is important to choose an appropriate method for the purpose at hand because each has both strengths and limitations and there is no such thing as a perfect method (Coulter et al. 2009).

Various patterns tend to recur frequently in the results of patient surveys, including the fact that younger people tend to be more critical of health services than older people and women are more critical than men (Zaslavsky et al. 2000). Studies have also found systematic differences between the views

Table 2.1 Quantitative and qualitative feedback methods

Quantitative	Qualitative
Self-completion postal surveys	In-depth face-to-face interviews (may be audio or video-taped)
Interviewer-administered face-to-face surveys	'Discovery' interviews carried out by clinical staff
Telephone surveys using live interviewers	Focus groups
Automated telephone surveys (interactive voice response – IVR)	Web-based feedback using free text comments
Online surveys using web-based or email questionnaires	Comment cards or suggestion boxes
Surveys using hand-held portable devices (PDAs or tablets) (on-site)	Video boxes (on-site)
Surveys on touch-screen kiosks (on-site)	Complaints and compliments
Surveys on bedside consoles (on-site)	Patient diaries
Administrative data/routine statistics	Mystery shopping and observation

of the public (healthy people/potential patients) and the views of current users of health services (Appleby and Rosete 2003). Those with recent experience as patients tend to give more positive reports about the NHS than the population as a whole. This disjunction between patients' and citizens' views is a paradox that takes some explaining. Some have suggested that public opinion polls asking for views on the NHS actually tap into more general views on the government of the day, picking up fluctuating political opinions (Mulligan and Appleby 2001). Those who are unhappy with the government for one reason or another may feel that all public services under their stewardship must be substandard.

Perceptions of NHS care

The influence of the media is often blamed for negativity, with television and newspapers tending to focus on adverse events that give a biased picture of the true state of the health service. Others have pointed out that NHS staff are themselves sometimes quite critical of the service and their employers (Edwards 2006). In a service that employs more than a million staff, their influence on public attitudes can be quite significant. Members of the public without recent NHS experience hear the horror stories and assume that these give an accurate picture of the service as a whole, while patients who have had good experiences that run counter to wider public perceptions may feel they have just been lucky.

Of particular concern is the fact that people from minority ethnic groups tend to report worse experiences than patients from the majority white population (Raleigh et al. 2004). Many of these differences remain significant after adjusting for variables such as age, sex and health status. While it is possible that some of the variation might be accounted for by different expectations or language difficulties, it seems likely that there are real differences in the experience of the different population groups that require further investigation and action.

Despite the fact that considerable resources are invested in measuring patients' experience using various feedback methods, the evidence that it leads to improvements in the quality of care is disappointingly thin. For example, the Care Quality Commission's patient surveys are widely noted by NHS organizations and undoubtedly help to focus attention on patients' experience, but the fact that the national results show little improvement year-on-year suggests that the act of measurement alone is insufficient to stimulate widespread change.

Incentivizing quality improvements

Systematic feedback can be helpful as a way of focusing attention on patients' experiences and initiating quality improvement programmes, but provider organizations may require additional help and stronger incentives to implement changes. A number of barriers to change have been identified (Davies and Cleary 2005):

- lack of incentives to change traditional ways of providing care
- lack of a patient-centred culture and values
- competing priorities
- lack of an effective quality improvement infrastructure
- lack of experience in focusing on patient interaction as a quality issue
- lack of relevant training and support
- lack of expertise in interpreting survey data
- lack of timely and specific results
- uncertainty about effective interventions or time frames for improvement
- perceived low cost-effectiveness of data collection
- scepticism, defensiveness and resistance to change.

Factors that can help to overcome these barriers include committed and engaged leadership from the board, senior clinicians and managers; regular monthly or quarterly feedback reports; an organization-wide approach with strong quality improvement structures; adoption of clear, focused goals; involvement of patients and families; and financial incentives (Davies et al. 2008). Patients' experience is related to staff attitudes to their jobs. An association has been noted between reports from staff on the organizational barriers and facilitators they experience in delivering care, and reports from patients on the quality of care received (Raleigh et al. 2009). This underlines the importance of managerial support, good working conditions and positive staff morale in providing a good experience for patients.

Pay-for-performance incentives have been introduced in a number of countries to stimulate quality improvements. For example, the UK's Quality and Outcomes Framework provides incentives for general practitioners to perform various evidence-based clinical procedures designed to enhance patient care. In 2008, in an attempt to strengthen the focus on patients' experience, the Department of Health in England announced the introduction of financial incentives for both general practices and hospitals linked to patient survey results (Secretary of State for Health 2008). There is evidence that these can be effective. In California, pay-for-performance incentives linked to primary care patient surveys led to significant improvements in communication and care coordination and physicians with lower baseline performance on patient experience measures experienced the largest improvements (Rodriguez et al. 2009). This type of financial stimulus might prove more effective than other attempts to improve patients' experience, but whether it will translate to a British setting remains to be seen.

Giving patients a choice of provider

Efforts to promote competition between providers (choice) have been used alongside patient feedback as a mechanism for change (voice). These aim to promote improvements by empowering patients to act as discerning consumers of healthcare. The idea is that people should be able to access comparative information on the quality of care available in different organizations (hospital or general practice), allowing them to select the best. Since payments follow the choices that patients make in a competitive healthcare market, in theory providers should have an incentive to improve the quality of their services in order to attract them.

While choice of provider has been the main focus of political attention in recent years, there are in fact many types of choices that appeal to patients, some of which may be of higher priority than provider choice (Figure 2.2) (Coulter 2010).

Historically there has been a trade-off in national health systems between cost-control and the amount of choice offered to patients (Bevan et al. 2010). Countries that fund healthcare out of taxation and those where access to hospital specialists requires a referral from a general practitioner (e.g. the UK and Denmark) have been relatively successful at controlling expenditure, but patient choice has been limited. On the other hand, those countries where funding is derived from social insurance (e.g. France and Germany) have allowed patients to go to any specialist of their choice but cost control has been more problematic. There are now signs that these distinctions are blurring, with the first group of countries introducing greater choice, and the second placing restrictions on choice by introducing various forms of

Choice of:
- Insurer, commissioner or payer of healthcare
- General practice (single-handed/group/polyclinic)
- Hospital (location/general/specialist)
- Provider type (NHS/private/voluntary sector)
- Access arrangements (general practice/walk-in centre/emergency department/helpline/online advice)
- Appointment time (including extended hours)
- Care location (hospital, community clinic or home)
- Type of professional (doctor, nurse, therapist)
- Specialist (including named doctors)
- Treatment (involvement in decisions)
- Care package (for long-term conditions)
- End-of-life care (place of death, when to cease active treatment, palliative care)

Figure 2.2 Types of healthcare choices

GP gatekeeping. A survey carried out among population samples in eight European countries, including the UK, found strong support for the notion of free choice of provider: 85 per cent wanted to be able to choose which specialist to see, and 86 per cent wanted a free choice of hospital (Coulter and Magee 2003). British people were among the most dissatisfied with the opportunities for making healthcare choices in their country, with only 30 per cent saying that these were 'good' or 'very good', compared to 73 per cent in Spain and 70 per cent in Switzerland.

Choice of general practitioner is the norm in most European countries, but there are often geographical limits to the choices on offer (Thomson and Dixon 2006). British patients have been able to choose which general practice to register with since the establishment of the NHS in 1948, albeit within tightly defined geographical limits, but until recently they had little say about who they were referred to for specialist advice or treatment. This changed in 2000 with the publication of the NHS Plan for England, which included a promise to give patients more choice (Secretary of State for Health 2000). Following a number of pilot projects, choice at the point of referral was introduced from December 2005. The choice on offer was essentially a choice of referral location, rather than a choice of individual specialist, and a new website, NHS Choices (www.nhs.uk) was set up to publish information on hospital quality indicators to inform people's choices. In 2008 the available choices were extended to include any hospital in the country, including private hospitals, and a legal right to choose was enshrined in the NHS Constitution. In March 2010, in a pre-election move, the Labour government launched a public consultation on extending choice in primary care by removing practice boundaries, with an intention to implement this nationally by April 2011. The coalition government that took over in May 2010 indicated its intention to proceed with this plan.

The pros and cons of choice

Critics of the policy – and there were many – claimed that it would lead to increased privatization, fragmentation and inefficiency, that it pandered to a middle-class agenda and that only those who were better off would benefit, leaving those in disadvantaged groups with few options. Barriers to access for these groups might include travel costs, job constraints, communication problems and low levels of health literacy. Since the availability of alternative providers is constrained in some regions and in some specialties, certain groups must be willing to travel long distances to take advantage of the offer of choice.

The government hoped that once patients were free to choose where to go, providers would have a strong incentive to drive up quality standards because funding flows would match the choices that patients made. Prices were fixed through a standard national tariff to ensure that competition was based on quality not cost, because price competition often leads to lower-quality standards. They expected commissioners (primary care trusts and budget-holding general practice groups) to establish arrangements to enable all eligible patients to exercise informed choices if they so wished, arguing that this was a way to reduce inequalities by opening up choice to those who had been denied it in the past (Stevens 2003). Pilot studies of patients offered a choice while on the waiting list for elective surgery had demonstrated that the offer of a choice of treatment location was popular and uptake was high. When patients waiting for cardiac surgery were offered the choice of going to another hospital with a shorter waiting list, about half of them opted to do so, sometimes travelling long distances (Le Maistre et al. 2004). Similarly, a high proportion (67 per cent) of patients in London awaiting a variety of elective surgical procedures opted for alternatives to their local hospital when given the choice (Coulter et al. 2005). There was no evidence of socio-economic differences in uptake in these pilots. Patients often weighed up a complex combination of factors to arrive at the decision that felt best for them, considering factors such as their present health status, waiting times, travel arrangements, convenience for family and friends, and where they would be likely to receive the best treatment and care. However, one of the most startling findings from the London Patient Choice pilot study was that over two thirds (68 per cent) of those eligible for the scheme were not offered the option of going to an alternative hospital, pointing to a reluctance on the part of clinicians and/or managers to encourage choice.

The debate about provider choice centres on its impact on quality, service development, equity and patient empowerment (see Table 2.2) (Coulter 2010). Many people have argued passionately for and against the policy on the basis

Table 2.2 Arguments for and against provider choice

Domain	For	Against
Quality	Leads to better patient experience, safety and clinical effectiveness	Increases fragmentation, reduces continuity, undermines population-based services
Service development	Improves access, increases plurality of providers, encourages innovation	Increases privatisation, destabilising existing NHS providers
Efficiency	Drives down costs, increases value-for-money	Increases transactions costs, requires spare capacity so is wasteful
Equity	Gives benefits of choice to those currently disadvantaged and disempowered	Increases inequalities because disadvantaged people can't take advantage of choice; choice isn't feasible in rural areas
Patient empowerment	Enhances patients' influence and improves responsiveness	Many patients don't want to choose; patients won't travel; increases demand to unsustainable levels

Source: Reproduced from Coulter (2010) with permission from the BMJ Publishing Group Ltd

of their expectations of its effects, but there is limited research evidence to confirm or refute the claims.

Exercising choice

Despite government enthusiasm for choice, surveys in England show that patients' awareness of the right to choose and GPs' willingness to offer a choice have been slow to grow (Dixon 2009). Four years after the scheme was supposed to have been implemented nationally, only half of eligible patients were aware that they could choose a provider and less than half of those referred said they had been offered a choice. Most patients are keen on having a choice, even if they choose to remain at their local hospital, but many GPs remain ambivalent or antagonistic to the idea (Dixon et al. 2010).

The offer of choice is popular among patients in all social strata, with older people, people with low educational qualifications, and those from mixed or non-white backgrounds being especially likely to value choice (Dixon et al. 2010). However, it is not clear that people want to spend time seeking out information to make their choices (Marshall and McLoughlin 2010). To date most patients have tended to rely on informal information sources, such as their GP's opinion, that of family and friends, or their own experience, with very few basing their decisions on officially published data on quality and performance. Even in the USA, where choice and competition has been integral to healthcare for many years, there is little evidence that patients' choices are influenced by published performance data (Fung et al. 2008). Nor is it evident that provider choice *per se* drives up quality standards. However, the fact that performance data are now publicly available does seem to have had an impact on providers, in some cases stimulating them to implement quality improvements (Friedberg et al. 2010). Since most patients do not use the information to shop around, it seems unlikely that these improvements were driven by financial incentives. Professional pride and managerial targets may be the key, stimulated by a desire to maintain parity with best practice benchmarks.

Strengthening patients' rights

Most developed countries and many less developed ones have passed laws to protect and promote patients' rights. These are often enshrined in patients' charters or bills of rights, setting out the obligations of healthcare organizations and staff towards service users. What these contain varies according to the legal framework of the country, the healthcare system, and social, cultural and ethical values, but there are certain themes that are common to patients' charters in different European countries (WHO Europe 1994):

- Everyone has the right to receive such healthcare as is appropriate to his or her health needs.
- Everyone has the right to health protection, disease prevention and the opportunity to pursue his or her highest attainable level of health.
- Everyone has a right to self-determination, to privacy and to respect.
- Patients must be fully informed about their health status and treatment options unless they explicitly say they do not want this information.
- Informed consent is a prerequisite for any medical intervention and for participation in research.
- All information about individual patients must be kept confidential.
- Patients have a right to high-quality care, continuity, dignity and respect.
- Patients have a collective right to be represented in the planning and evaluation of health services.

Patients' rights legislation was a phenomenon of the 1990s (Coulter 2002). Throughout the decade many countries introduced laws or charters to clarify these rights. That this legislation was considered necessary was an interesting reflection on changing attitudes to healthcare – a sign that people had become less willing to trust health professionals to safeguard their interests. The charters were intended as a means of drawing attention to patients' rights, thereby strengthening them and setting down standards that could be publicly monitored.

The Patients' Charter

The first UK patients' charters (for England, Wales and Scotland) were introduced in 1991, but the English charter was subsequently revised in 1995 and 1997. While helpful in the sense of raising awareness and setting standards, the legislation did not necessarily advance patients' legal rights as much as it might have appeared. Although they used the language of rights, most of these took the form of general statutory duties rather than legally enforceable individual entitlements. The first patients' charter was introduced by a Conservative government and it set various targets that healthcare providers were expected to achieve, including waiting time targets which had been the subject of great public concern. When they came to power in 1997 the new Labour government commissioned a review of the Patient's Charter. This was critical of the way it had been implemented and of its unintended consequences (Dyke 1998). Many NHS staff resented the fact that the charter had been imposed on them by the government. They had not been consulted about its development and hence were not fully committed to achieving the goals it set. They saw it as a stick to beat them with and they felt it led to a distortion of priorities, particularly the guaranteed minimum waiting times. They also felt the charter encouraged unrealistic expectations without placing obligations or responsibilities on patients themselves.

Following this review, the government promised to replace the Patient's Charter with a new charter that would emphasize patients' responsibilities as well as their rights and would include a guide for the public on how to access health services. When it finally appeared in 2001, the new version was very different from the original charter (Department of Health 2001). All mention of 'rights' had been expunged, to be replaced by 'commitments', 'responsibilities' and 'expectations'. The new approach was intended to look more like a contract between the NHS and its users than a charter and it seemed more designed to reassure staff than to empower patients. However, waiting time targets were strengthened and huge efforts were made to achieve them. Patients requiring hospital treatment were promised a maximum wait of 18 weeks from referral to treatment and, following a coordinated effort led by the Department of Health and pressure on managers to achieve the target, in 2008 the government was able to claim success (Secretary of State for Health 2008). The policy drew vociferous complaints from some quarters because the centrally imposed targets were felt to have had a distorting effect on clinical priorities. There was no doubting the fact that single-minded pursuit of targets had driven down waiting times dramatically, but there were some unintended consequences. Most serious of these was the fact that it encouraged an obsession with hospital treatment at a time when the government was trying to move more care out of hospitals into the community.

The NHS Constitution

A further shift in direction occurred in 2009 with the publication of the NHS Constitution (Department of Health 2009). This reinstated the language of 'rights' to set out the legal commitments to patients (i.e. those that were backed by legislation), and 'pledges' that the NHS was expected to achieve. Patients' responsibilities were enumerated (e.g. the need to register with a GP, to keep appointments, and to participate in public health programmes), as were the rights and responsibilities of staff. This time NHS organizations were placed under a legal obligation to have regard to the NHS Constitution in all their decisions and actions and to monitor compliance.

Charters or constitutions have a potentially important role in improving the quality of care, but their effects depend on how they are implemented, monitored and enforced. This must be done with care, with efforts made to engage stakeholder representatives in their development, publicizing them effectively to staff and patients, rigorously monitoring outcomes and offering redress when standards fall short. They must be backed up by an effective complaints system, with local resolution where possible, and access to independent review when necessary. Unless all these mechanisms are in place they risk being seen simply as window-dressing that can safely be ignored by staff and dismissed as irrelevant by patients.

Involving patients in redesigning services

It seems clear that measuring patients' experiences, giving them more choice and publicizing their rights can help to promote quality improvement, but these initiatives on their own are not enough to ensure that services are truly patient-centred. What else can be done?

There are numerous theories on how to implement change in an organization. These have been usefully summarized by Richard Grol and his colleagues who reviewed the following approaches to organizational change (Grol et al. 2005):

- theories of innovative organizations
- theory of quality management
- process re-engineering theory
- complexity theory
- theory of organizational learning
- theories of organizational culture
- economic theories.

The learning from these different theoretical approaches has been distilled to produce an integrated model for implementing change in healthcare (Grol and Wensing 2005) (Figure 2.3).

The model is intended to be helpful for planning and executing specific improvements. Patients and carers can be involved throughout the process, or in specific parts of it, and patient feedback can be used both as the starting

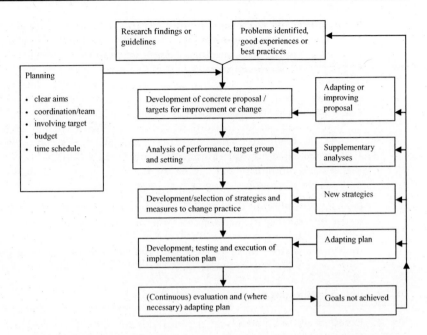

Source: Reproduced with permission from Grol and Wensing (2005, Figure 3.1, p. 45)

Figure 2.3 Implementation of change: a model

point and for monitoring progress. However, maintaining improvements year-on-year can pose additional challenges. The process is not always as neat and linear as implied in the model.

For example, a study of six US academic medical centres highlighted the importance of cultural change in sustaining improvements in patients' experience (Shaller and Darby 2009). The six hospitals were engaged in a process of implementing patient and family-centred care across their organizations. These organizations described the process they went through as a journey. The journey was triggered by entirely different events in each organization, never followed a straight line, was led at different levels in the organization and moved at different paces. Nevertheless, it was possible to identify six core elements of a successful change strategy that were common to all the hospitals:

- **Visionary leadership:** Each organization was characterized by strong, visionary leadership committed to achieving the goals of patient and family-centred care.
- **Dedicated champion:** A dynamic, dedicated champion was responsible for driving necessary changes at the operational level.

- **Partnerships with patient and families:** Active collaboration with patients and families was central to the change strategy on multiple levels, including policy and planning, patient care and medical education.
- **Focus on the workforce:** Principles of patient and family-centred care were incorporated into human resource policies and determined the way staff were recruited, trained and rewarded.
- **Effective communication:** Clear communication at every level, from board to management to front-line workers to patients and families helped spread and reinforce patient and family-centred values and procedures.
- **Performance measurement and monitoring:** Continuous measurement and monitoring were necessary to assess progress and identify new opportunities for improving performance.

Other organization-level strategies that are likely to be important include leadership training and development, training in quality improvement concepts and methods, rewards and incentives, and examples of evidence-based tools and initiatives that have been shown to work well in other settings.

Experience-based design

Experience-based design is an approach developed by the NHS Institute for Innovation and Improvement to help health professionals understand patients' experience and respond appropriately (Bate and Robert 2008). Drawing on theories from anthropology and design science, it aims to draw out the subjective, personal feelings a patient or carer experiences at crucial points in the care pathway and use these to develop insights and opportunities for improvement. It does this by:

- Encouraging and supporting patients and carers to 'tell their stories'.
- Using these stories to pinpoint those parts of the care pathway where the users' experience is most powerfully shaped (the 'touchpoints').
- Working with patients, carers and front-line staff to redesign these experiences rather than just systems and processes.

Involvement of patients and carers is central to the process, both for illuminating the problems and co-designing the solutions. It draws on various techniques, including semi-structured questionnaires, narrative analysis and customer journey mapping to produce detailed process maps identifying the emotional highs and lows experienced by patients during an episode of care. Then all those involved – staff and patients or carers – examine the process and discuss how the experience could be improved. Further measurement can be used to monitor changes. Adopted by a number of NHS organizations, this approach can prompt anything from small-scale changes to care processes up to major service redesign.

This question of whether patient involvement makes service redesign more effective has not been adequately addressed in research to date. A systematic review that tried to address the question found 337 studies about involving patients in the planning and development of healthcare, but only 13 per cent of these described the effects of involvement and most of these used case study design instead of more rigorous comparative or experimental methods (Crawford et al. 2002). The review described improvements in patient information, improved appointment procedures, extended opening times, improved transport arrangements, and better access for people with disabilities, and new services that had been developed in response to patients' requests; for example, advocacy services, employment opportunities, complementary treatments, crisis services and fertility treatments. There were also reports of the abandonment or modification of plans to close hospitals as a result of listening to public concerns. Despite this, the authors of the review drew attention to the complexity of the topic and difficulties involved in attributing specific changes to the fact that patients and public were involved.

The precise effects of patient participation on the quality and effectiveness of services are unclear at present, but it is important to remember that absence of evidence must not be mistaken for absence of effect. It would be misleading to conclude that a particular course of action is ineffective, just because it has not been thoroughly researched.

Summary

This chapter has outlined various initiatives designed to promote greater responsiveness to patients' needs and experiences. Specifically we have focused on how policy levers such as 'voice' and 'choice' might be used to incentivize improvements in the quality of care. Various definitions of 'patient-centred care' have been noted, together with the different methods for measuring this concept. We have seen that measurement will not be sufficient to create improvements unless there are additional triggers to stimulate action. One potential trigger is to encourage patients to review the performance of healthcare providers and use this information to choose where to go for advice or treatment. Another is to involve both patients and professionals more directly in redesigning services. Publicizing patients' rights and monitoring standards may also help, especially if these are reinforced by financial incentives. Various theories have been invoked to inform the planning of quality improvement strategies, but achieving the necessary cultural change can be difficult. There is still a great deal to learn about the best way to stimulate improvements in healthcare delivery.

References

Appleby, J. and Rosete, A.A. (2003) The NHS: keeping up with public expectations? In A. Park et al. (eds), British Social Attitudes: The 20th Report – Continuity and Change over Two Decades (pp. 29–43). London: Sage Publications.
Bate, P. and Robert, G. (2008) Bringing User Experience to Healthcare Improvement: The Concepts, Methods and Practices of Experience-based Design. Oxford: Radcliffe Publishing.

Berwick, D.M. (2009) What 'patient-centered' should mean: confessions of an extremist, *Health Aff (Millwood)*, 28(4): 555–65.

Bevan, G., Helderman, J.K. and Wilsford, D. (2010) Changing choices in health care: implications for equity, efficiency and cost, *Health Economics, Policy Law*, 5(3): 251–67.

Brady, C. and Frampton, S.B. (2009) Breaking down the barriers to patient-centred care, in S.B. Frampton and P. Charmel (eds). *Putting Patients First: Best Practices in Patient-centred Care* (pp. 285–300). San Francisco, CA: Jossey Bass.

Coulter, A. (2002) *The Autonomous Patient*. London: The Nuffield Trust.

Coulter, A. (2006) *Engaging Patients in their Healthcare: How is the UK Doing Relative to Other Countries?* Oxford: Picker Institute Europe.

Coulter, A. (2010) Do patients want a choice and does it work?, *British Medical Journal*, 341: c4989.

Coulter, A. and Magee, H. (2003) *The European Patient of the Future*. Maidenhead: Open University Press.

Coulter, A., Fitzpatrick, R. and Cornwell, J. (2009) *Measures of Patients' Experience in Hospital: Purpose, Methods and Uses*. London: King's Fund.

Coulter, A., Le Maistre, N. and Henderson, L. (2005) *Patients' Experience of Choosing Where to Undergo Surgical Treatment: Evaluation of the London Patient Choice Scheme*. Oxford: Picker Institute.

Crawford, M.J., Rutter, D., Manley, C., Weaver, T., Bhui, K., Fulop, N. and Tyrer, P. (2002) Systematic review of involving patients in the planning and development of health care, *British Medical Journal*, 325(7375): 1263.

Davies, E. and Cleary, P.D. (2005) Hearing the patient's voice? Factors affecting the use of patient survey data in quality improvement, *Quality and Safety in Health Care*, 14(6): 428–32.

Davies, E., Shaller, D., Edgman-Levitan, S., Safran, D.G., Oftedahl, G., Sakowski, J. and Cleary, P.D. (2008) Evaluating the use of a modified CAHPS survey to support improvements in patient-centred care: lessons from a quality improvement collaborative, *Health Expectations*, 11(2): 160–76.

Delbanco, T., Berwick, D.M., Boufford, J.I., Edgman-Levitan, S., Ollenschlager, G., Plamping, D. and Rockefeller, R.G. (2001) Healthcare in a land called PeoplePower: nothing about me without me, *Health Expectations*, 4(3): 144–50.

Department of Health (2001) *Your Guide to the NHS*. London: Department of Health.

Department of Health (2009) *The NHS Constitution*. London: Department of Health.

Dixon, J. and Alakeson, V. (2010) *Reforming Health Care: Why We Need to Learn from International Experience*. London: The Nuffield Trust.

Dixon, A., Robertson, R., Appleby, J., Burge, P., Devlin, N. and Magee, H. (2010) *Patient Choice: How Patients Choose and How Providers Respond*. London: The King's Fund.

Dixon, S. (2009) *Report on the National Patient Choice Survey March 2009*. London: Department of Health.

Dyke, G. (1998) *The New NHS Charter – A Different Approach*. London: Department of Health.

Edwards, N. (2006) *Lost in Translation: Why are Patients More Satisfied with the NHS than the Public?* London: NHS Confederation.

Friedberg, M.W., Steelfisher, G.K., Karp, M. and Schneider, E.C. (2010) Physician groups' use of data from patient experience surveys, *Journal of General Internal Medicine*, DOI:10.1007/S11606-010-1597-1.

Fung, C.H., Lim, Y.W., Mattke, S., Damberg, C. and Shekelle, P.G. (2008) Systematic review: the evidence that publishing patient care performance data improves quality of care, *Annals of Internal Medicine*, 148(2): 111–23.

Grol, R. and Wensing, M. (2005) Effective implementation: a model, in R. Grol, M. Wensing, and M. Eccles (eds) *Improving Patient Care: The Implementation of Change in Clinical Practice* (pp. 41–70). Oxford: Elsevier.

Grol, R., Wensing, M., Hulscher, M. and Eccles, M. (2005) Theories on implementation of change in healthcare, in R. Grol, M. Wensing and M. Eccles (eds), *Improving Patient Care: The Implementation of Change in Clinical Practice* (pp. 15–40). Oxford: Elsevier.

Haynes, R.B., Ackloo, E., Sahota, N., McDonald, H.P. and Yao, X. (2008) Interventions for enhancing medication adherence, *Cochrane Database of Systematic Review*. 2: CD000011.

Institute of Medicine (2001) *Crossing the Quality Chasm: A New Health System for the 21st Century*. Washington, DC: National Academy Press.

Keating, N.L., Green, D.C., Kao, A.C., Gazmararian, J.A., Wu, V.Y. and Cleary, P.D. (2002) How are patients' specific ambulatory care experiences related to trust, satisfaction, and considering changing physicians?, *Journal of General Internal Medicine* 17(1): 29–39.

Le Grand, J. (1999) Competition, cooperation, or control? Tales from the British National Health Service, *Health Aff (Millwood)* 18(3): 27–39.

Le Maistre, N., Reeves, R. and Coulter, A. (2004) *Patients' Experience of CHD Choice*. Oxford: Picker Institute Europe.

Marshall, M. and McLoughlin, V. (2010) How do patients use information on health providers?, *British Medical Journal* 341: c5272.

Mead, N. and Bower, P. (2000) Patient-centredness: a conceptual framework and review of the empirical literature, *Social Science and Medicine* 51(7): 1087–1110.

Meterko, M., Wright, S., Lin, H., Lowy, E. and Cleary, P.D. (2008) *Mortality Among Patients with Acute Myocardial Infarction: The Influences of Patient-centred Care and Evidence-based Medicine*. Oxford: Picker Institute.

Mulligan, J. and Appleby, J. (2001) The NHS and Labour's battle for public opinion, in A. Park et al. (eds), *British Social Attitudes* (18th Report edn.) London: Sage Publications.

Patients Association (2009) *Patients Not Nmbers, People Not Statistics*. London: Patients Association.

Raleigh, V.S., Hussey, D., Seccombe, I. and Qi, R. (2009) Do associations between staff and inpatient feedback have the potential for improving patient experience? An analysis of surveys in NHS acute trusts in England, *Quality and Safety in Health Care*, 18(5): 347–54.

Raleigh, V.S., Scobie, S., Cook, A., Jones, S., Irons, R. and Halt, K. (2004) *Unpacking the Patients' Perspective: Variations in NHS Patient Experience in England*. London: Commission for Health Improvement.

Richards, N. and Coulter, A. (2007) *Is the NHS Becoming More Patient-centred? Trends from the National Surveys of NHS Patients in England 2002–07*. Oxford: Picker Institute Europe.

Rodriguez, H.P., von, G.T., Elliott, M.N., Rogers, W.H. and Safran, D.G. (2009) The effect of performance-based financial incentives on improving patient care experiences: a statewide evaluation, *Journal of General Internal Medicine*, 24(12): 1281–88.

Schoen, C., Osborn, R., How, S.K., Doty, M.M. and Peugh, J. (2009) In chronic condition: experiences of patients with complex health care needs, in eight countries, 2008, *Health Aff (Millwood)* 28(1): w1–16.

Schoen, C., Osborn, R., Squires, D., Doty, M.M., Pierson, R. and Applebaum, S. (2010) How health insurance design affects access to care and costs, by income, in eleven countries, *Health Aff (Millwood)*, 29(12): 2323–34.

Secretary of State for Health (2000) *The NHS Plan: A Plan for Investment, a Plan for Reform*. London: The Stationery Office.

Secretary of State for Health (2008) *High Quality Care for All: NHS Next Stage Review Final Report*. London: Department of Health.

Shaller, D. and Darby, C. (2009) *High-performing Patient and Family-centered Academic Medical Centers: Cross-site Summary of Six Case Studies*. Camden, ME: Picker Institute Inc.

Spence, A. (2010) *Social Trends: International Comparisons*. London: Office for National Statistics, Social Trends 41.

Stevens, S. (2003) Equity and choice: can the NHS offer both? A policy perspective, in A. Oliver (ed.). *Equity in Health and Healthcare*. London: The Nuffield Trust.

The Mid Staffordshire NHS Foundation Trust Inquiry (2010) *Independent Inquiry into Care Provided by Mid Staffordshire NHS Foundation Trust January 2005–March 2009*. London: The Stationery Office.

Thomson, S. and Dixon, A. (2006) Choices in health care: the European experience, *Journal of Health Services Research and Policy*, 11(3): 167–71.

Wensing, M., Jung, H.P., Mainz, J., Olesen, F. and Grol, R. (1998) A systematic review of the literature on patient priorities for general practice care. Part 1: Description of the research domain, *Social Science and Medicine*, 47(10) 1573–88.

World Health Organization (WHO) Europe (1994) *A Declaration on the Promotion of Patients' Rights in Europe*. Copenhagen: World Health Organization.

Zaslavsky, A.M., Zaborski, L. and Cleary, P.D. (2000) Does the effect of respondent characteristics on consumer assessments vary across health plans?, *Medical Care Research Review*, 57(3): 379–94.

Further reading

Bate, P. and Robert, G. (2007) *Bringing User Experience to Healthcare Improvement: The Concepts, Methods and Practices of Experience-based Design*. Oxford: Radcliffe Publishing.

Calnan, M. and Rowe, R. (2008) *Trust Matters in Health Care*. Maidenhead: Open University Press.

Frampton, S. B. and Charmel, P. (2009) *Putting Patients First: Best Practices in Patient-centred Care*. San Francisco, CA: Jossey-Bass.

Green, S. (2007) *Involving People in Healthcare Policy and Practice*. Oxford: Radcliffe Publishing.

Grol, R., Wensing, M. and Eccles, M. (2005) *Improving Patient Care: The Implementation of Change in Clinical Practice*. Oxford: Elsevier.

Institute of Medicine (2001) *Crossing the Quality Chasm: A New Health System for the 21st Century*. Washington, DC: National Academy Press.

Tritter, J., Daykin, N., Evans, S., and Sanidas, M. (2004) *Improving Cancer Services through Patient Involvement*. Abingdon: Radcliffe Medical Press.

3 Building health literacy

3

Overview

In this chapter we consider health literacy and its fundamental importance in strategies to improve health, reduce inequalities and engage patients and the public. Topics covered include defining and measuring health literacy, the theory and practice of health education, health information for the public and its quality and reliability, media coverage of health and healthcare, and use of the media and social marketing to disseminate health messages.

The importance of health literacy

Health literacy is the ability to read, understand and act upon health information. The US Institute of Medicine defines it as follows:

> The degree to which individuals have the capacity to obtain, process, and understand basic health information and services needed to make appropriate health decisions.
>
> (Institute of Medicine 2004: 32)

While this definition emphasizes the relevance of health literacy to clinical care, health literacy is also fundamental to public health. With that in mind Don Nutbeam has proposed a broader definition:

> A set of capacities that enable individuals to exert greater control over their health and the range of personal, social and environmental determinants of health.
>
> (Nutbeam 2008, presentation)

The concept includes listening and speaking (oral literacy), reading and writing (print literacy) and numeracy, but it also includes basic health knowledge and the cognitive ability to understand and use this to make health-related decisions. Health literacy is essential for good health. If people cannot obtain, understand and use health information, they will not be able to look after themselves effectively, navigate the health system without difficulty, or make appropriate health choices for their own, their family and their community's health.

Functional skills of literacy and numeracy are an essential component of health literacy. People who struggle with reading, writing and arithmetic are likely to have lower levels of basic health knowledge, impeding their ability to interpret symptoms or engage in health promoting or self-care behaviour. They may find it more difficult to read and understand relevant instructions such as how to take prescribed medicines; and they often face greater problems in understanding and communicating with health professionals. However, health literacy is much more than being able to read and understand health information. It is also about the competence to make health decisions. As such it is relevant to the whole population, not just those with low basic literacy and numeracy skills.

Three levels of health literacy can be distinguished (Nutbeam 2000):

1 **Functional**: basic skills in reading and writing for understanding health information.
2 **Interactive**: more advanced cognitive and social skills to enable active participation in healthcare choices.
3 **Critical**: the ability to analyse health information critically and make effective use of it.

Literacy and health inequalities

Improving health literacy is critically important in tackling health inequalities. Research by the Institute of Medicine in the USA found that people with low health literacy:

• had poorer health status
• experienced more hospital admissions
• were less likely to adhere to treatment recommendations
• experienced more drug and treatment errors
• made less use of preventive services (Institute of Medicine 2004).

A review commissioned by the American Medical Association concluded that health literacy was a stronger predictor of health status than age, income, employment status, education level, race or ethnic group, but disentangling cause and effect is tricky (Ad Hoc Committee on Health Literacy 1999). While low health literacy is strongly associated with poor health, it is also related to poverty, unhealthy lifestyles and other social determinants of health (DeWalt et al. 2004).

Measuring health literacy

Measuring levels of health literacy can be problematic. Different studies have used various different measures and indicators of literacy and numeracy, but these focus mainly on testing people's ability to read and understand instructions and do not extend to more complex issues such as effective oral communication or empowerment. Nevertheless, it is clear that efforts to improve health and increase patient engagement must include finding ways to overcome health literacy barriers.

There has been less attention to the topic in the UK than in North America, but levels of functional health literacy were assessed among a UK population sample in a 2007 study. This used a simple test of the ability to read and understand materials that patients might encounter in health settings (e.g. instructions for taking medicines and eligibility for exemption from prescription charges) (von Wagner et al. 2007). The results suggested that around 11 per cent of adults struggled with these basic tasks. Those with poor literacy skills were more likely to be:

- older
- male
- lower educational attainment
- lower income
- worse diet
- less exercise
- smokers
- worse self-rated health.

In fact the problem may be even worse than the UK study suggested. More extensive surveys in other countries have found greater proportions of people who lack the basic literacy, numeracy and health knowledge skills required to make sensible decisions about their health and healthcare. For example, studies in the USA have found that around a quarter of patients could not understand medication instructions or information about appointment times and a very pessimistic Canadian study concluded that 60 per cent of adult Canadians lacked the capacity to make informed health decisions (Berkman et al. 2004; Murray et al. 2007).

Even people with good basic literacy and numeracy skills may struggle to understand and interpret health information in a way that prompts them to act appropriately to protect or enhance their health. While tackling low levels of health literacy requires carefully developed approaches targeted at those with special needs, it is also important to address the health information needs of the whole population. Because health literacy is central to enhancing involvement of patients in their care, all strategies designed to strengthen patient engagement should focus on improving health literacy.

Raising standards

Health literacy is the outcome of a complex array of individual, social and economic processes, but improving people's understanding of their health is seen as fundamental for improving health outcomes. The Institute of Medicine has identified three broad factors that contribute to health literacy, each of which constitutes a potential intervention point: culture and society (shared ideas, meanings, values, attitudes and beliefs), the education system (including adult and professional education), and the health system and all those who work within it (Institute of Medicine 2004).

Responsibility for improving standards of health literacy rests within all these sectors, but those working in the health system have a very important role to play, with considerable potential to make a difference. Patients look to them to provide information about their health and to educate them in how to manage illness and long-term conditions. This is recognized in professional standards which underscore the professional's responsibility to inform and educate. For example, the General Medical Council's standards for doctors, set out in *Good Medical Practice,* require them to share with patients, in a way they can understand, the information they want or need to know about their condition, its likely progression, and the treatment options available to them, including associated risks and uncertainties (General Medical Council 2006). Doctors are also enjoined to respond to patients' questions, to keep them informed about the progress of their care, and to make sure, wherever practical, that arrangements are made to meet patients' language and communication needs.

Similarly, the Nursing and Midwifery Council tells its members:

> You must recognise and respect the contribution that people make to their own care and wellbeing. You must make arrangements to meet people's language and communication needs. You must share with people, in a way they can understand, the information they want or need to know about their health.
>
> (Nursing and Midwifery Council 2008, standards 10, 11, 12)

Building health literacy is a key underpinning for initiatives that aim to improve public health. Of course the major determinants of ill-health are socio-economic, environmental and political, and there are limits to what individuals can do alone (Wilkinson and Pickett 2010). Nevertheless, helping people to understand the factors that shape their health is an important function for health systems. Responsibility for promoting public health lies within many sectors of public and commercial life and spans the responsibilities of many government departments, but the NHS and all those who work within it have a clear and important role to play.

Health education

Educational approaches to improve levels of health literacy among disadvantaged groups take many forms, including courses for small groups, formal education in schools, colleges and adult education institutions and one-to-one counselling. Skilled for Health is one such example. A national programme run by the Department of Health in England, together with the Department for Business Innovation and Skills and ContinYou, a learning and health charity, the programme aimed to help people improve their health while boosting their language, literacy and numeracy skills. Educational sessions on a range of health topics, such as healthy eating, exercise and first aid, were delivered to people in deprived areas. An integral part of efforts to tackle health inequalities, the programmes were intended to provide useful information and skills and improve people's confidence to look after their health. An internal evaluation of the second phase of the programme found that retention rates were high, with 84 per cent of 3,000 learners completing the programme, and 25 per cent of these going on to register for further courses (ContinYou 2010). Participants' health knowledge increased significantly, particularly in the areas of healthy eating, exercising, smoking, drinking and looking after their mental health, with benefits also accruing to their families and communities.

People's capability to manage their own health can be improved. Judith Hibbard, a researcher at the University of Oregon, has developed a tool for measuring people's level of activation; in other words, their capacity for managing their own health. Patient activation involves four stages: (1) believing the patient role is important; (2) having the confidence and knowledge necessary to take action; (3) actually taking action to maintain and improve one's health, and (4) staying the course even under stress (Hibbard et al. 2004). Patients with high scores on the patient activation measure (PAM) are better at self-managing their health than those with low scores and achieve better health outcomes (Mosen et al. 2007). A survey of a UK population sample found that only 22 per cent of those aged 45 and over were confident that they could manage their health effectively at times of stress (Ellins and Coulter 2005).

A survey of clinicians based in the UK and the USA found that many were unwilling to support patient activation (Hibbard et al. 2010). They were much more likely to agree that patients should follow medical advice than that they should make independent judgements or take independent actions. The good news is that it appears possible to intervene to improve people's ability to manage their health by carefully targeting interventions to their activation level, increasing the likelihood of better health outcomes (Hibbard et al. 2009).

Theories of health behaviour

When designing, implementing and evaluating educational initiatives such as these, it is important to take account of theories of health behaviour. These can help with categorizing and explaining people's behaviour and itemizing the steps involved in making changes. They can also illuminate the environmental or contextual factors that influence the way people behave and learn. Most theories of health behaviour that inform health education are cognitive-behavioural; that is, they start from the following three premises (National Cancer Institute 2005):

1 Behaviour is mediated by cognitions; in other words, what people know and think affects how they act.
2 Knowledge is necessary for, but not sufficient to produce, most behaviour changes.

3 Perceptions, motivations, skills, and the social environment are key influences on behaviour.

The theories operate at three different levels – individual, interpersonal and community. Individual and interpersonal theories are focused on changing people's behaviour, while community theories incorporate strategies to change the environment. Fishbein has produced a combined or integrative model that includes the main elements from each of the most commonly referenced theories (Figure 3.1) (Fishbein 2009).

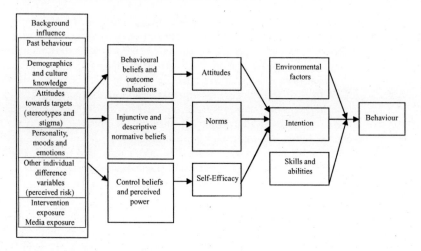

Source: Reproduced from Fishbein (2009) with permission from John Wiley & Sons, Inc.

Figure 3.1 Integrative model of behavioural prediction

The integrative model is based on the idea that people's behaviour follows reasonably from their beliefs. The key elements of health-related behaviour include attitudes and motivation, normative influences or social pressure, and a person's self-efficacy or abilities and confidence, all of which are influenced by their background beliefs. Interventions to change behaviour must take account of each of these influences. Since health literacy is closely related to self-efficacy, improving people's knowledge, understanding and skills is likely to be a necessary component of an intervention to promote health, but it may not be sufficient unless environmental factors and intentions to change are also tackled.

Theory-based or not, robust evidence on the effectiveness of educational interventions in reducing the health gap between socio-economic groups is hard to find. Studies have tended to measure health knowledge as the primary outcome, with mixed results (Pignone et al. 2005). It is of course possible to improve levels of health knowledge and understanding among people with low levels of health literacy, but relying on educational programmes on their own is not usually an effective way to improve health. For example, despite the fact that group educational programmes are routinely provided for pregnant women, there is very little evidence that the effects of these extend beyond minor knowledge gains and social contact with other mothers, which in itself can be useful but is unlikely to impact on health inequalities (Gagnon and Sandall 2007).

Educational sessions may work better if they are combined with other measures; for example, the use of simplified written materials, graphics, videos or other audio-visual materials, together with personalized support and reminders. However, while there is some evidence that more complex interventions can improve people's knowledge and confidence, there is very little evidence that this leads to better health outcomes (Clement et al. 2009).

Part of the problem lies in the fact that educational programmes have tended to use traditional didactic methods that may not be well received by people who struggled with these when they were at school. Directive styles of teaching and advice-giving tend to generate resistance or a sense of hopelessness in those on the receiving end. More engaging methods may prove more successful, such as motivational interviewing (Rollnick et al. 2010). Rollnick and colleagues recommend the following communication strategies to motivate behaviour change:

- Use a guiding rather than a directive style – ask open-ended questions, listen to the person's account and reflect it back in a brief summary, exchange information and discuss it.
- Elicit the person's own motivation to change – discuss what they want to change, the pros and cons of changing behaviours, how important they feel it is to change and how confident they feel.
- Help the person to set and monitor their own goals, encourage and support them in achieving and, if necessary, modifying these.

A systematic review of 72 studies found that using motivational interviewing to stimulate healthy behaviours worked much better than traditional advice-giving (Rubak et al. 2005). The authors argued for a shift of emphasis 'from monologue to dialogue' between patients and healthcare providers, with much greater emphasis on encouraging patients to determine their own goals for behaviour change rather than complying with the professional's agenda.

Despite years of experience of health education, there are still wide gaps in our knowledge of what works best. Carefully targeted interventions can lower health risks among disadvantaged groups, but the extent to which they reduce inequalities between groups with different levels of literacy, or between different socio-economic groups, has not been well studied.

Health information

Most strategies for tackling health literacy across the whole population, as opposed to those targeted at specific population groups, have focused on improving the provision of health information. Good quality health information is essential for patient involvement in healthcare. Patients and the public require information that is timely, relevant, reliable and easy to understand. This is an essential component of any strategy to support self-care, shared decision-making, self-management of long-term conditions and health promotion. Patients have many decisions to make about their healthcare and, like all decision-makers, they require information to inform their choices. Reliable information is also essential to help people understand their health problems and how to deal with them. Good quality health information is needed for various reasons:

- to understand what is wrong
- to gain a realistic idea of prognosis
- to choose a provider
- to make the most of consultations
- to understand the processes and likely outcomes of tests, treatments, services
- to participate in care and treatment decisions
- to assist in self-care/self-management.

Health information is ubiquitous. You can find it in leaflets, magazines, books, radio and television programmes and on the Internet. Yet many people complain that finding the right information at the right time is very difficult. Insufficient information about their illness and its treatment is the most common problem identified in patient surveys.

Information sources

For most patients the first and most trusted information source is their doctor, although many also seek out supplementary information from a variety of sources. A telephone survey carried out with a national random sample of the UK population in 2005 asked respondents (n = 3,000) where they looked for health information: the majority (80 per cent) said they were likely or very likely to seek out information to learn about how to cope with health problems (Ellins and Coulter 2005). Nearly three-quarters said they would expect their doctor to provide it, but a wide variety of other sources were also mentioned (Figure 3.2).

Certain groups are more likely to be active information-seekers. Younger people see themselves as more informed than the previous generation and many no longer regard the medical profession as the fount of all knowledge. They are more likely to be familiar with Internet search techniques and often seek alternative sources of health information, not necessarily because they distrust the doctor but because they are used to checking out information from a variety of sources before making major decisions.

There are some exceptions to this trend: for example, patients with serious conditions may be fearful of finding more information in case it contains

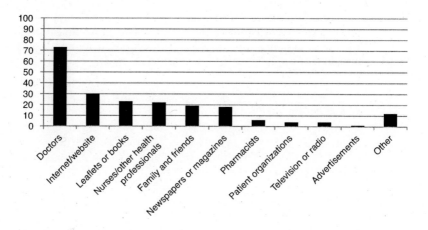

Source: Ellins and Coulter (2005).

Figure 3.2 Sources of health information

bad news. Women tend to be more active information-seekers than men, and people with chronic illnesses and parents with children at home often go to considerable lengths to obtain health information. Many people find that exchange of experiences with other patients or ex-patients is the most reassuring and efficient way to get information.

Many people look to health professionals to signpost them to reliable information about local services, but they are often disappointed when clinicians do not systematically or proactively provide this information (Swain et al. 2007). For their part health professionals often feel threatened when patients bring information they have found on the Internet to a consultation, despite the fact that most patients see this as a helpful resource to support valued relationships, not a challenge to their authority (Ahluwalia et al. 2010; Stevenson et al. 2007). Health professionals often fail to anticipate patients' information needs and do not offer information proactively; instead, they leave patients to extract it by asking the right questions of the right person at the appropriate time – a tall order for many.

Health information on the Internet

The Internet is increasingly used as a source of health information, particularly by younger and more educated people. It has been calculated that around the world each day, more than 12.5 million health-related computer searches are conducted on the World Wide Web (Eysenbach 2003). People welcome the opportunity it gives for quick access to information from anywhere in the world, but many find the quantity of health websites overwhelming and tracking down reliable information takes considerable time and effort (Coulter and Magee 2003). A systematic review of 79 studies evaluating the quality of Internet health information found many problems: about a third of nearly 6,000 websites assessed were found to contain information that was inaccurate (Eysenbach et al. 2002).

The extent to which people are motivated to understand their health problems is an even more important predictor of Internet use than demographic factors. People who believe that access to information will enable them to deal better with their health will go to considerable lengths to obtain relevant information and use is highest among those with Internet access at home (Mead et al. 2003). The British government's public facing health website, NHS Choices, attracts seven million users each month and there is some evidence that it changes their health behaviour, reducing the demand for GP consultations (Nelson et al. 2010). A majority of UK households now has Internet access – the figure rose to 19.2 million households in 2010, 73 per cent of the total, ranging from 59 per cent in North East England to 83 per cent in London, with 31 per cent of Internet users connecting via mobile phones (Office for National Statistics 2010). Sixty per cent of adults in the UK use the Internet every day or almost every day. This gives a very large pool of people who are likely, at some time or another, to search the Internet for health information. The increasing uptake of mobile broadband, accessible via smartphones, with applications enabling direct access to health websites, will further increase this trend.

The information needs of those without Internet access must not be forgotten. This currently amounts to more than a quarter of the adult population. Despite the rapid spread of Internet access, surveys suggest that a persistent minority will remain excluded from the digital revolution for some time to come. According to one survey, about one in ten people said their main reason for not having Internet access was because of its cost, while 13 per cent said they were not interested in having it and could not see what they would do with it if they did (MORI 2009). Most other people without Internet access have plans to get it in the near future.

Although use of the Internet by people aged over 65 is growing fast, they are still much less likely to use it than those in younger age groups. Sixty per cent of UK adults aged 65 and over had never used the Internet, compared with 22 per cent of those aged between 55 and 64 and just 1 per cent of 16–24-year-olds (Office for National Statistics 2010). People from lower socio-economic groups are also less likely to be regular Internet users. These groups tend to make proportionally greater use of telephone helplines when they need information and advice on health issues (Ellins and Coulter 2005).

Information quality

There have been a number of initiatives designed to clarify the needs of information users and improve the quality of health information, including guidelines and checklists. Information quality checklists are usually based on a combination of ethical standards and research evidence (Coulter et al. 2006). Most of these stress the importance of the characteristics listed in Table 3.1.

Table 3.1 Quality criteria for health information

1. Clear purpose	The information product clearly explains its aims and purpose
2. Relevant links	The material meets a clearly defined need and has been tested with representatives of the target audience; where possible to sources of further information and support are provided
3. Evidence-based	The information is consistent with up-to-date clinical evidence, medical and social research; personal opinion is clearly distinguished from evidence-based information
4. Authoritative	Sources of evidence are clearly indicated; names and credentials of authors, funders and sponsors are clearly stated; any conflict of interest is disclosed; any advertising is clearly identified
5. Complete	Where relevant, all alternative treatment, management or care options are clearly stated and all possible outcomes are clearly presented
6. Secure	Where users' personal details are requested, there is a clear policy for safeguarding privacy and confidentiality
7. Accurate	The product has been checked for accuracy; in the case of user generated content there is a clear procedure for moderation
8. Well-designed	The layout is clear and easy to read; if necessary, the product contains specific navigation aids such as content lists, indexing and search facilities
9. Readable	The language is clear, where possible conforming to recognized plain language standards and available in minority languages where relevant
10. Accessible	There is a clear dissemination plan for the product; the material conforms to accepted standards for accessibility, where possible including versions for use by people with sensory and learning difficulties
11. Up-to-date	The date of issue or latest update is clearly indicated along with the planned review date

Attempts to ensure that health information matches up to these quality standards have used accreditation schemes to signpost reliable information and incentivize information producers. For example, the Health on the Net Foundation launched its voluntary certification scheme in 1996. Run by a not-for-profit foundation based in Geneva, by 2010 it had certified more than

6,800 health websites in 118 countries. In 2009 the Department of Health in England launched a similar scheme to accredit health information producers. Known as the Information Standard (www.theinformationstandard.org), the scheme was designed to ensure that health and social care information for patients, carers and members of the public is accurate, impartial, balanced, appropriately researched, accessible and well written. Information producers who achieve certification can put the Information Standard's logo on their publications or websites as a sign that the production process meets the standard and their information products are trustworthy. The success of such schemes depends on the extent to which they help people find reliable information and whether they help to improve information quality. Published evidence that they achieve these goals is hard to find.

Information as therapy

There is no shortage of health information, but it is not well signposted. There is a lack of coordination between information providers and until recently it was rare to find a local organization acting as a central information point, collating and providing information about the range of health and social care services in a locality (Swain et al. 2007). The situation is beginning to improve as the growing use of information technology in healthcare offers opportunities to embed patient information into clinical systems so that it can be much more readily accessed and used.

It is now possible for electronic health information systems to automatically 'prescribe' specially targeted information to be printed out in the clinic, GP surgery or community pharmacy, or sent by email, secure messaging or telephone, based on information in patients' electronic medical records. In developing the concept of 'information therapy', in which information is seen as directly beneficial to health in the same way as prescribing medicines or other treatments, Kemper and Mettler (2002) described three approaches to improving the delivery of health information:

1 **Physician-prescribed information therapy**: Information prescriptions made directly by a health professional based on their knowledge of the patient and the medical decisions he or she faces.
2 **System-prescribed information therapy**: Health information systems automatically 'push' targeted information to the patient based on what the system knows about the patient's decision-making needs.
3 **Consumer-prescribed information therapy**: Well-designed search systems allow patients to find information themselves, either through direct searches or by referral from self-help groups, family members or friends.

Impact of health information

The impact of patient information crucially depends on the context and way in which it is used. While much health information is intended to be accessed and used directly by patients, carers or members of the public, without mediation by health professionals, many information producers hope that their information products will supplement and reinforce professional advice rather than replace it. Indeed, health professionals have a key role in ensuring that patients are able to access, understand and make appropriate use of information resources. Without such support, patients may feel confused by what they read or face difficulties relating it to their own circumstances, reducing the impact of the information.

The provision of written and electronic information meets an important felt need. It can help to increase patients' sense of empowerment, improving their coping ability and helping to reduce anxiety. For example, it has been estimated that about 39 per cent of those with cancer in developed countries use the Internet to find information or support (Eysenbach 2003). They may use it to obtain information about prognosis or treatment recommendations, or to communicate with other patients as a form of 'virtual' support. An overview of 24 surveys with responses from more than 8,000 cancer patients suggested that this type of knowledge and support can be helpful for increasing their sense of confidence and self-efficacy and helping to reduce the loneliness that sufferers can experience (Eysenbach 2003).

There is evidence that good-quality information materials, both printed and electronic, can improve patients' knowledge and understanding of their condition, including those with low health literacy (RTI International 2004). The impact is greater when written information is tailored to the individual and reinforced by verbal information from clinicians (Johnson et al. 2003). This would appear to be a more useful strategy than simply leaving leaflets in the general practice waiting room or including them in packaging. The leaflets that are found in pill packets comply with legal requirements imposed by the regulators, but studies have found that they do not meet patients' medicine information needs adequately, nor is there any evidence that they help to improve adherence to medicine-taking regimes (Haynes et al. 2008; Raynor et al. 2007). Improving the design of these leaflets might help to reduce medication errors (Ioannidis and Lau 2001). Web-based information may contribute to improvements in health behaviours when used as part of a well-designed educational programme. Some studies have suggested that web-based interventions could be more effective at stimulating behaviour change than more traditional information sources (Wantland et al. 2004).

Health in the media

Newspapers, magazines and broadcast media are the main means by which we keep informed about what is going on in the world beyond our immediate environment and they are an influential source of information about health and healthcare. Medical and health features are very popular and can be found in every newspaper and in most broadcasting schedules. People's response to this information can influence the lifestyle choices they make, the decisions they take when they are ill, the health professionals they choose to consult, and their willingness to accept the advice or treatment offered. In responding to public interest in these issues, the print and broadcast media play an important part in shaping public expectations.

The influence of the mass media can be both benign and malign, providing useful information that educates and informs, but also on occasions promulgating inaccurate or biased stories that mislead, confuse or alarm (Coulter 2004). Journalists, television producers and editors are obliged to be selective in their choice of topics. Their choices, or news values, are governed largely by their knowledge of their readership or audience and their interests. This knowledge also influences the way in which the information is presented. Writing about medical news stories in British radio and television programmes, Karpf distinguished seven types of story which featured regularly:

- the breakthrough (scientific discoveries leading to potential new treatments)
- the disaster (health consequences of earthquakes, fires, explosions, or accidents)
- the ethical controversy (e.g. surrogate mothers, test-tube babies)
- the scandal (e.g. deaths from prescribed drugs, violence by psychiatric patients)
- the strike (health service dispute or political debate)
- the epidemic (its course and treatment)
- the official report or speech (government or medical) (Karpf 1988).

This categorization still fits the majority of health news items, although the amount of attention given to each will vary over time, depending on factors such as the extent of political interest in specific healthcare issues.

In selecting what to write about and what to publish, journalists and editors are influenced by the characteristics of the newspaper or television channel, the source of the story and the availability of specialist expertise, competition from other types of story or feature, interest from other media outlets, and their intuition and views on 'newsworthiness'. Much news is 'manufactured', in the sense that it is generated by organizations and interests external to the news media to suit a particular purpose. Conscientious journalists do not usually reproduce press releases uncritically without looking for alternative interpretations, but the news agenda is largely shaped by those who have a particular interest in influencing public opinion. And of course not all journalists and editors are conscientious or scrupulous in their quest for the truth. The views of large institutions, public bodies and commercial corporations tend to dominate because they can afford to invest in press and public relations departments whose job is to influence the media. In the health arena these can include industrial or commercial interests, such as the pharmaceutical industry or insurance companies, political parties, government departments, professional organizations and voluntary groups (Entwistle and Sheldon 1999).

This means that the public is bombarded with health information of varying quality and reliability, much of which represents the views of particular vested interests. Studies have shown that the news media tends to present a biased and overly optimistic picture of the benefits of medical care, with information about harms and side-effects played down and alternative or cheaper treatments not mentioned (Schwitzer 2008). Specialist health journalists writing in broadsheet newspapers do a significantly better job than non-specialists, but falling revenues from traditional media mean that these specialisms are under threat (Wilson et al. 2010). In the meantime, many of those with low health literacy get their information about health and medical treatments from media outlets that do not employ well-informed specialist journalists.

Television drama and features programmes cover health topics too and these can also influence public attitudes. Drama series such as *ER*, *Casualty*, *Holby City* and *House MD* provide viewers with behind-the-scenes stories which help to shape expectations of real-life health professionals and institutions. Although many such programmes strive for realism, the requirements of drama, including programme length and narrative pace, ensure that the picture they present is a distorted one.

Impact of media stories

Evidence on the impact of media stories on health behaviour presents a complex picture. Stories that provoke alarm can lead people to take action, sometimes with adverse consequences. For example, press coverage of research linking oral contraceptive use with an increased risk of venous thromboembolism scared some women into giving up effective contraception, leading to an increase in the numbers seeking abortion (Drife 2001). Parental concern about adverse publicity surrounding childhood vaccinations for pertussis in the 1970s and MMR in the 1990s resulted in reduced immunization rates and an increase in the incidence of serious childhood illnesses (Nicoll et al. 1998). In both cases, media reports of research studies had failed to emphasize the cautious nature of the researchers' conclusions, focusing instead on raising alarm about the implied risks.

There is also evidence that the mass media can have a positive effect on health behaviour, and many health education campaigns have incorporated media publicity as a key component (Wakefield et al. 2010). For example, well-designed media campaigns have succeeded in achieving small reductions in the number of young people who take up smoking (Sowden and Arblaster 2000). In the Netherlands, a mass media campaign on the use of folic acid to reduce the risk of neural tube defects increased awareness and use of folic acid among pregnant women (de Walle et al. 1999). In Switzerland in 1984, extensive media publicity about excessive and rising hysterectomy rates in Canton Ticino led to a reduction of a third in the use of this operation (Domenighetti et al. 1988). A British campaign to reduce the stigma associated with depression employed newspaper and magazine articles, radio and television programmes, leading to significant positive changes in attitudes (Paykel et al. 1998).

A systematic review of the effects of mass media interventions on health service utilization identified 17 studies, 14 of which evaluated formal campaigns and three looked at media coverage of health-related issues (Grilli et al. 2002). All but one concluded that mass media coverage was effective in promoting beneficial change, including uptake of immunization and cancer screening, education about HIV risk, and reducing delay in admission to hospital for patients with suspected myocardial infarction. Media campaigns to change health behaviour seem to work best if they are carefully targeted and sustained, and accompanied by linked interventions, such as the availability of practical support (Wakefield et al. 2010).

Disease-mongering

Pharmaceutical companies and other commercial bodies that produce treatments, medical devices or diagnostic equipment have an interest in promoting demand for their products. Direct-to-consumer advertising of prescribed medical products is banned in every developed country except the USA and New Zealand, so the companies use other means, such as feature articles in newspapers and magazines, or 'disease-awareness' campaigns, to get their message across. They have shown themselves adept at getting publicity for their products by encouraging feature stories, some of which have had a profound effect on demand. The publication in 1990 of a prominent article about Prozac in the international news magazine *Newsweek* resulted in widespread publicity in many European news media and a dramatic increase in sales of the drug (Nelkin 1996). Similarly, the anti-impotence drug Viagra became a news sensation throughout the world. This type of free publicity carries the risk that it can increase demand for inappropriate medical interventions, potentially causing harm to patients and increasing pressure on scarce health resources. In some cases it involves persuading healthy people that they have a condition that could benefit from treatment, a process that has been dubbed 'disease-mongering' (Moynihan et al. 2002).

Companies claim that their disease-awareness campaigns provide useful public education, helping to draw attention to unrecognized or untreated conditions. It is indeed the case that many health problems go unrecognized in their early stages – for example diabetes, hypertension, osteoporosis or raised cholesterol – when early diagnosis and treatment may be beneficial. In addition, people sometimes suffer health problems that they are reluctant to consult their doctors about, either because of the embarrassing nature of the condition or because they do not know that effective treatments are available: examples include incontinence and impotence. Other common problems, such as male-pattern baldness, obesity or social anxiety may not be perceived as medical in nature, yet medications are now available which could help some sufferers.

The case for increasing public awareness of methods to prevent disease progression or making it more acceptable to seek help for embarrassing problems may have considerable force, but it does not follow that responsibility for tackling this should be delegated to commercial companies. To allow companies to make the running in public education results in a stress on those, often minor, conditions for which there is a branded pharmaceutical product and medicalization of normal life processes. Evidence from the USA, where this type of advertising or advertorial is sanctioned, shows that commercial interests can often lead to scare-mongering (Mintzes 2002).

Healthy people are encouraged to think they need medical attention by the use of alarming imagery, or statistics quoted out of context; for example, suggesting that minor memory lapses might be the first sign of Alzheimers disease, or citing a one in two chance of having osteoporosis leading to broken bones and dowager's hump. Pharmaceutical companies, often working in alliance with doctors and patient groups, have aimed to show that ordinary processes or ailments are medical problems (e.g. baldness), that mild symptoms might be portents of serious disease (e.g. irritable bowel syndrome), that personal or social problems can be redefined as medical problems (e.g. social phobia), that risk factors can be reconceptualized as diseases (e.g. osteoporosis), and that disease prevalence is greater than it really is (e.g. erectile dysfunction).

Improving public education about disease and treatment is an appropriate public health goal, but it is not a good idea to relax the advertising restrictions to achieve this, as the companies would like governments to do. Doing so would result in a distortion of priorities to suit commercial ends and would do nothing to educate the public about the limitations of medical care. Pharmaceutical companies often complain that they know more about their products than anyone else yet they are uniquely subject to restrictions on imparting this information. They point to the large amount of unreliable health information now available on the Internet, some of which may be more harmful than properly regulated drug advertisements. In Europe the industry has been lobbying the European Commission to allow patients to access information about their products on their websites. It is argued that this would meet patients' needs for more information and would help improve compliance with medicine-taking. However, there is no evidence that the type of information that companies would provide would have any impact on compliance. Advertisements tend to be superficial in their coverage of medical conditions and their treatments. They seldom educate patients about how the drug works, its relative effectiveness, alternative treatments, or behavioural changes that could augment or supplant drug therapy. Information produced by the commercial sector is the least trusted of any information source (Coulter et al. 1998). People want unbiased information from independent sources that they can trust; promotion information about individual products will not meet this need.

What is needed is a concerted effort to make evidence-based patient information much more widely available, coupled with public education to help people critically appraise medical information. Health literacy is important, not just because of the contribution it could make to improving health behaviours, but also as a defence against commercial pressures promoting expensive products that may not benefit people's health.

Social marketing

As we have seen, the popular media can have a benign as well as a malign effect on health. They can be a useful vehicle for public education about health and illness and systematic marketing techniques using various types of mass media can be used to promote behaviour that benefits people's health or encourage them to consume products that harms it.

Government departments and health authorities are among those who aim to use the mass media to promote particular health messages using social marketing techniques. Social marketing has been defined as:

> ... the systematic application of marketing alongside other concepts and techniques, to achieve specific behavioural goals for a social good.
>
> (French and Blair-Stevens 2007: 1)

Social marketing for public health aims to help people make healthy choices, adopt healthier lifestyles or make better use of health services. French and his colleagues have described eight characteristics of social marketing (Table 3.2) (French et al. 2009).

Drawing on experience from the commercial sector as well as on health promotion techniques developed by public sector and voluntary organizations, social marketing is increasingly seen by governments and public bodies as the method of choice for engaging people in health improvement. It is essentially a more systematic approach to health promotion using tried and tested techniques, often on a larger scale than have been attempted in the past, and informed by commercial insights (e.g. segmentation, marketing theory) and theories of behaviour change.

Since social marketing advocates using several interventions at the same time in pursuit of a health improvement goal, it is quite hard to measure its impact. Evaluative research is easier to do when the topic of the study is a single, well-defined intervention carried out in controlled conditions. Monitoring the effects of complex, multifaceted projects is much more demanding and the results are unlikely to be clear-cut.

The task is not impossible, however. Four reviews of the effectiveness of social marketing approaches came to the following conclusions (Stead and Gordon 2010):

1 **Nutrition**: social marketing can be an effective way to increase fruit and vegetable intake, reduce fat intake, and improve dietary knowledge, and can have a positive influence on attitudes to healthy eating, but

Table 3.2 Characteristics of social marketing

1. Customer orientation	Develops a robust understanding of the audience, based on market and consumer research, combining data from different sources
2. Behaviour and behavioural goals	Focuses on achieving impact on specific aspects of people's behaviour, and understands the factors that shape behaviour
3. Theory based	Draws on behavioural theory to inform and steer development, taking account of physical, psychological, social, environmental and economic influences
4. Insight	Aims to develop a deeper 'insight' into people's lives, with a strong focus on what will move and motivate people
5. Exchange	Recognizes costs to the target audience(s) (financial, physical, social, time spent) and perceived benefits
6. Competition	Ensures that all those things competing for the time, attention, and behaviour of the audience are addressed
7. Segmentation	Uses demographic, epidemiological and social data to 'segment' the target audience and tailor messages to their specific needs
8. Methods mix	Uses an appropriate mix of interventions to achieve the goals

Source: Reproduced from French et al. (2009) with permission from Oxford University Press

few studies showed an effect on physiological variables such as blood pressure, cholesterol or body mass index.

2 **Substance misuse**: social marketing can reduce smoking, alcohol consumption and illicit drug use among young people, but it is less successful at encouraging smoking cessation in the general population.

3 **Physical activity**: the effects of social marketing interventions on exercise rates appear to be mixed, with some evidence of a positive effect on walking frequency among middle-aged people and positive effects on exercise-related knowledge, but very little effect on general physical activity or physiological outcomes.

4 **Workplace interventions**: some promising effects on employees' health and well-being, particularly from intensive interventions, but sustaining participation was a challenge.

There is still much to learn about the best ways to engage people in health improvement. Social marketing is a promising approach and since it aims to build knowledge and empower people to take action, its success rests on its impact on health literacy in the target populations.

Summary

Health literacy involves more than just the ability to read and understand health information. It also includes interpreting probabilities and having the confidence to make health decisions. All strategies that aim to strengthen patient engagement and reduce health inequalities should include a focus on improving health literacy. Educational approaches are more effective when they take account of theories of health behaviour. These help to explain people's behaviour and the steps involved in making changes. Providing health information that is tailored to people's needs is a key element in improving health literacy and this should conform to recognized quality standards. The media can have both a malign and a benign influence on health beliefs. Awareness of its effects can be turned to good use in social marketing campaigns which can be effective as a means of empowering people to make healthy choices.

References

Ad Hoc Committee on Health Literacy (1999) Health literacy: report of the Council on Scientific Affairs, American Medical Association, *Journal of the American Medical Association*, 281(6): 552–57.

Ahluwalia, S., Murray, E., Stevenson, F., Kerr, C. and Burns, J. (2010) 'A heartbeat moment': qualitative study of GP views of patients bringing health information from the Internet to a consultation, *British Journal of General Practice*, 60(571): 88–94.

Berkman, N.D., DeWalt, D.A., Pignone, M.P., Sheridan, S.L., Lohr, K.N., Lux, L., Sutton, S.F., Swinson, T. and Bonito, A.J. (2004) Literacy and health outcomes, *Evidence Reports/Technology Assessments*, 87: 1–8.

Clement, S., Ibrahim, S., Crichton, N., Wolf, M. and Rowlands, G. (2009) Complex interventions to improve the health of people with limited literacy: a systematic review, *Patient Education and Counseling*, 75(3): 340–51.

ContinYou (2010) *Skilled for Health has 'the Heineken Effect'*. Coventry: ContinYou.

Coulter, A. (2004) Medicine and the media, in R. Jones et al. (eds), *Oxford Textbook of Primary Medical Care* (pp. 107–11). Oxford: Oxford University Press.

Coulter, A. and Magee, H. (2003) *The European Patient of the Future*. Maidenhead: Open University Press.

Coulter, A., Ellins, J., Swain, D., Clarke, A., Heron, P., Rasul, F., Magee, H. and Sheldon, H. (2006) *Assessing the Quality of Information to Support People in Making Decisions about their Health and Healthcare*. Oxford: Picker Institute Europe.

Coulter, A., Entwistle, V. and Gilbert, D. (1998) *Informing Patients: An Assessment of the Quality of Patient Information Materials*. London: King's Fund.

de Walle, H.E., van der Pal, K.M., de Jong-van den Berg, L.T., Jeeninga, W., Schouten, J.S., de Rover, C.M., Buitendijk, S.E. and Cornel, M.C. (1999) Effect of mass media campaign to reduce socioeconomic differences in women's awareness and behaviour concerning use of folic acid: cross sectional study, *British Medical Journal*, 319(7205): 291–92.

DeWalt, D.A., Berkman, N.D., Sheridan, S., Lohr, K.N. and Pignone, M.P. (2004) Literacy and health outcomes: a systematic review of the literature, *Journal of General Internal Medicine*, 19(12): 1228–39.

Domenighetti, G., Luraschi, P., Casabianca, A., Gutzwiller, F., Spinelli, A., Pedrinis, E. and Repetto, F. (1988) Effect of information campaign by the mass media on hysterectomy rates, *The Lancet*, 2(8626–27): 1470–73.

Drife, J.O. (2001) The third generation pill controversy ('continued'), *British Medical Journal*, 323: 119–20.

Ellins, J. and Coulter, A. (2005) *How Engaged are People in their Healthcare? Findings of a National Telephone Survey*. Oxford: Picker Institute.

Entwistle, V. and Sheldon, T. (1999) The picture of health? Media coverage of the health service, in B. Franklin (ed.), *Social Policy, the Media and Misrepresentation* (pp. 118–34). London: Routledge.

Eysenbach, G. (2003) The impact of the Internet on cancer outcomes, *CA Cancer Journal for Clinicians*, 53(6): 356–71.

Eysenbach, G., Powell, J., Kuss, O. and Sa, E.R. (2002) Empirical studies assessing the quality of health information for consumers on the world wide web: a systematic review, *Journal of the American Medical Association*, 287(20): 2691–700.

Fishbein, M. (2009) An integrated model for behavioral prediction and its application to health promotion, in R.J. DiClemente, R.A. Crosby and M.C. Kegler (eds), *Emerging Theories in Health Promotion Practice and Research* (pp. 215–34). San Francisco, CA: Jossey–Bass.

French, J. and Blair-Stevens, C. (2007) *Big Pocket Book: Social Marketing*. London: National Social Marketing Centre.

French, J., Blair-Stevens, C., McVey, D. and Merritt, R. (2009) *Social Marketing and Public Health: Theory and Practice*. Oxford: Oxford University Press.

Gagnon, A.J. and Sandall, J. (2007) Individual or group antenatal education for childbirth or parenthood, or both, *Cochrane Database of Systematic Review*, no. 3, p. CD002869.

General Medical Council (2006) *Good Medical Practice*. London: GMC.

Grilli, R., Ramsay, C. and Minozzi, S. (2002) Mass media interventions: effects on health services utilisation, *Cochrane Database of Systematic Review*, 1: CD000389.

Haynes, R.B., Ackloo, E., Sahota, N., McDonald, H.P. and Yao, X. (2008) Interventions for enhancing medication adherence, *Cochrane Database of Systematic Review* 2: CD000011.

Hibbard, J.H., Collins, P.A., Mahoney, E. and Baker, L.H. (2010) The development and testing of a measure assessing clinician beliefs about patient self-management, *Health Expectations*, 13(1): 65–72.

Hibbard, J.H., Greene, J. and Tusler, M. (2009) Improving the outcomes of disease management by tailoring care to the patient's level of activation, *American Journal of Managed Care*, 15(6): 353–60.

Hibbard, J.H., Stockard, J., Mahoney, E.R. and Tusler, M. (2004) Development of the Patient Activation Measure (PAM): conceptualizing and measuring activation in patients and consumers, *Health Services Research*, 39(4): 1005–26.

Institute of Medicine (2004) *Health Literacy: A Prescription to End Confusion*. Washington, DC: The National Academies Press.

Ioannidis, J.P. and Lau, J. (2001) Evidence on interventions to reduce medical errors: an overview and recommendations for future research, *Journal of General Internal Medicine*, 16(5): 325–34.

Johnson, A., Sandford, J. and Tyndall, J. (2003) Written and verbal information versus verbal information only for patients being discharged from acute hospital settings to home, *Cochrane Database of Systematic Review*, 4: CD003716.

Karpf, A. (1988) *Doctoring the Media: The Reporting of Health and Medicine*. London: Routledge.

Kemper, D.W. and Mettler, M. (2002) *Information Therapy: Prescribed Information as a Reimbursable Medical Service*. Boise, ID: Healthwise Inc.

Mead, N., Varnam, R., Rogers, A. and Roland, M. (2003) What predicts patients' interest in the Internet as a health resource in primary care in England?, *Journal of Health Services Research and Policy*, 8(1): 33–39.

Mintzes, B. (2002) For and against: direct to consumer advertising is medicalising normal human experience: for, *British Medical Journal*, 324(7342): 908–9.

MORI (2009) *Accessing the Internet at Home*. London: Ofcom.

Mosen, D.M., Schmittdiel, J., Hibbard, J., Sobel, D., Remmers, C. and Bellows, J. (2007) Is patient activation associated with outcomes of care for adults with chronic conditions?, *Journal of Ambulatory Care Management*, 30(1): 21–29.

Moynihan, R., Heath, I. and Henry, D. (2002) Selling sickness: the pharmaceutical industry and disease mongering, *British Medical Journal*, 324(7342): 886–91.

Murray, S., Rudd, R., Kirsch, I., Yamamoto, K. and Grenier, S. (2007) *Health Literacy in Canada: Initial Results from the International Adult Literacy and Skills Survey*. Ottawa: Canadian Council on Learning.

National Cancer Institute (2005) *Theory at a Glance: A Guide for Health Promotion Practice*. Washington, DC: US Department of Health and Human Services, National Institutes of Health.

Nelkin, D. (1996) An uneasy relationship: the tensions between medicine and the media, *The Lancet*, 347: 1600–3.

Nelson, P., Murray, J. and Kahn, M.S. (2010) *NHS Choices Primary Care Consultation Final Report*. London: Imperial College.

Nicoll, A., Elliman, D. and Ross, E. (1998) MMR vaccination and autism 1998: deja-vu pertussis and brain damage 1974?, *British Medical Journal*, 316: 715–16.

Nursing and Midwifery Council (2008) *The Code: Standards of Conduct, Performance and Ethics for Nurses and Midwives*. London: Nursing and Midwifery Council.

Nutbeam, D. (2000) Health literacy as a public health goal: a challenge for contemporary health education and communication strategies into the 21st century, *Health Promotion International*, 15(3): 259–67.

Nutbeam, D. (2008) Health literacy: perspectives from Australia. Health Literacy Group. Available online at http://www.healthliteracy.org.uk/publications/148-health-literacy-perspectives-from-australia-don-nutbeam-nov-08.

Office for National Statistics (2010) Internet access 2010: households and individuals, Statistical Bulletin, Office for National Statistics, Southport.

Paykel, E.S., Hart, D. and Priest, R.G. (1998) Changes in public attitudes to depression during the Defeat Depression Campaign, *British Journal of Psychiatry*, 173: 519–22.

Pignone, M., DeWalt, D.A., Sheridan, S., Berkman, N. and Lohr, K.N. (2005) Interventions to improve health outcomes for patients with low literacy: a systematic review, *Journal of General Internal Medicine*, 20(2): 185–92.

Raynor, D.K., Blenkinsopp, A., Knapp, P., Grime, J., Nicolson, D.J., Pollock, K. et al. (2007) A systematic review of quantitative and qualitative research on the role and effectiveness of written information available to patients about individual medicines, *Health Technology Assessment*, 11(5): 1–160.

Rollnick, S., Butler, C.C., Kinnersley, P., Gregory, J. and Mash, B. (2010) Motivational interviewing, *British Medical Journal*, 340: 1242–45.

RTI International (2004) *Literacy and Health Outcomes*. Rockville, MD, 87. Agency for Healthcare Research and Quality.

Rubak, S., Sandbaek, A., Lauritzen, T. and Christensen, B. (2005) Motivational interviewing: a systematic review and meta-analysis, *British Journal of General Practice*, 55(513): 305–12.

Schwitzer, G. (2008) How do US journalists cover treatments, tests, products, and procedures? An evaluation of 500 stories, *PLoS Medicine*, 5(5): e95.

Sowden, A.J. and Arblaster, L. (2000) Mass media interventions for preventing smoking in young people, *Cochrane Database of Systematic Review*, 2: CD001006.

Stead, M. and Gordon, R. (2010) Providing evidence for social marketing's effectiveness, in J. French et al. (eds) *Social Marketing and Public Health: Theory and Practice* (pp. 81–96). Oxford: Oxford University Press.

Stevenson, F.A., Kerr, C., Murray, E. and Nazareth, I. (2007) Information from the Internet and the doctor-patient relationship: the patient perspective – a qualitative study, *BMC Family Practice*, 8: 47.

Swain, D., Ellins, J., Coulter, A., Heron, P., Howell, E., Magee, H., Cairncross, L., Chisholm, A. and Rasul, F. (2007) *Accessing Information about Health and Social Care Services*. Oxford: Picker Institute Europe.

von Wagner, C., Knight, K., Steptoe, A. and Wardle, J. (2007) Functional health literacy and health-promoting behaviour in a national sample of British adults, *Journal of Epidemiology and Community Health*, 61(12): 1086–90.

Wakefield, M.A., Loken, B. and Hornik, R.C. (2010) Use of mass media campaigns to change health behaviour, *The Lancet*, 376(9748): 1261–71.

Wantland, D.J., Portillo, C.J., Holzemer, W.L., Slaughter, R. and McGhee, E.M. (2004) The effectiveness of Web-based vs. non-Web-based interventions: a meta-analysis of behavioral change outcomes, *Journal of Medical Internet Research*, 6(4): e40.

Wilkinson, R. and Pickett, K. (2010) *The Spirit Level: Why Equality is Better for Everyone*. London: Penguin Books.

Wilson, A., Robertson, J., McElduff, P., Jones, A. and Henry, D. (2010) Does it matter who writes medical news stories?, *PLoS Medicine*, 7(9): e1000323.

Further reading

French, J., Blair-Stevens, C., McVey, D. and Merritt, D. (2010) *Social Marketing and Public Health: Theory and Practice*. Oxford: Oxford University Press.

Institute of Medicine (2004) *Health Literacy: A Prescription to End Confusion*. Washington, DC: The National Academies Press.

Kemper, D.W. and Mettler, M. (2002) *Information Therapy: Prescribed Information as a Reimbursable Medical Service*. Boise, ID: Healthwise.

Moynihan, R. and Cassells, A. (2005) *Selling Sickness: How the World's Biggest Pharmaceutical Companies Are Turning Us All Into Patients*. Vancouver: Greystone Books.

Wilkinson, R. and Pickett, K. (2010) *The Spirit Level: Why Equality is Better for Everyone*. London: Penguin Books.

4 Selecting treatments

Overview

This chapter introduces the concept of shared decision-making for clinical treatments, diagnostic tests, screening, prevention and condition management, and outlines various strategies for involving patients in decisions about their treatment and care and improving decision quality. These include the use of patient decision aids, techniques for communicating risk effectively, and advance care planning. The challenges involved in introducing these changes into clinical practice are outlined.

Shared decision-making

The most common source of patient dissatisfaction is not being properly informed about their condition and the options for treating it. Most patients want more information than they are routinely given by health professionals, and many would like a greater share in the process of making decisions about how to treat their health problems (Grol et al. 2000).

Shared decision-making is a process in which patients are involved as active partners with professionals in clarifying acceptable treatment, management or support options, discussing goals and priorities, and together planning and implementing a preferred course of action. It involves three key components:

1 Provision of reliable, balanced, evidence-based information outlining treatment options, outcomes and uncertainties.
2 Decision support counselling with a clinician or a health coach to clarify options and preferences.
3 A system for recording, communicating and implementing patients' preferences.

Shared decision-making is appropriate in any situation when there is more than one reasonable course of action and no one option is self-evidently best for everyone. This situation is very common since there are often many different ways to treat a health problem, each of which may lead to a different set of outcomes. In these cases it is important to spell out the options and what is known about the likely outcomes of each of these, and to encourage patients to say what is most important to them. These are known as 'preference-sensitive' decisions (O'Connor et al. 2007).

For example, a woman facing a decision on how to treat early stage breast cancer needs to know that it can be treated by removing only the tumour (lumpectomy) followed by radiotherapy, or by removing the whole breast (mastectomy) followed by plastic surgery to reconstruct the breast if she wishes to do this (Collins et al. 2009). The first option involves a less invasive procedure and may produce a better cosmetic result, but there is a slightly greater risk that the patient will need a second operation later. Plus she will have to attend the hospital for radiation treatment over a period of weeks, which can cause unpleasant side-effects. Mastectomy is a more major operation and the decision about reconstruction is not straightforward – there are different ways in which it can be done and some women dislike the thought of having a 'false' breast – but for some women the 'take it all away' option gives them greater peace of mind. The good news is that both mastectomy and lumpectomy plus radiotherapy produce equivalent results in terms of survival. So there is a genuine choice and the best course of action depends on how the woman feels about retaining or losing her breast, how she feels about the risk of requiring further surgery, and her attitudes to the inconvenience and discomfort of radiotherapy and the cosmetic effect of reconstruction. The doctor cannot make an appropriate treatment choice without eliciting the patient's preferences.

Other common examples of preference-sensitive choices include treatment for low back pain, prostate or ovarian cancer, benign uterine conditions, menopausal symptoms, hip and knee osteoarthritis, and screening for conditions such as prostate cancer or colorectal cancer (see Table 4.1).

Practice variations

In these and many other cases the patient's attitude to the likely benefits and risks should be a key factor in the decision. However, the evidence suggests that very few patients facing these types of decisions are fully informed about the key facts that should influence their selection of appropriate treatments, and attempts to elicit their informed preferences are relatively rare (Fagerlin et al. 2010; Zikmund-Fisher et al. 2010). In part this is because doctors have traditionally assumed the role of decision-maker, acting as the patient's agent to determine the most appropriate course of action. This would be justifiable if medicine was as scientific and evidence-based as it purports to be, but evidence of wide variations in practice patterns shows that many other factors influence decisions, in particular doctor's beliefs and preferences (Right Care 2010). These are not always rational and scientific or based on a clear understanding of the patient's situation and preferences.

Practice variations arise because many healthcare interventions have not been rigorously evaluated, or because the evidence that does exist is ignored; because of a prevailing view that 'more is better' allowing the supply of services to drive demand; and because health professionals fail to inform patients about the balance between benefits and harms and do not take

Table 4.1 Some examples of preference-sensitive treatment choices

Condition	Treatment options
Abnormal uterine bleeding	Watchful waiting Medications Medicated intrauterine device ((IUD) Endometrial ablation Hysterectomy
Benign prostatic hyperplasia	Watchful waiting Medication Prostatectomy Minimally invasive surgery
Coronary artery disease	Medications Angioplasty and stent insertion Bypass surgery
Early stage breast cancer	Mastectomy Lumpectomy Breast reconstruction Chemotherapy Hormone therapy
Knee osteoarthritis	Lifestyle changes (weight loss, exercise) Non-drug treatments (physiotherapy, shoe inserts, walking aids, knee braces, ice and heat) Pain medications Injections Complementary therapies Surgery (arthroscopy, osteotomy, knee replacement)
Menopause symptoms	Hormone replacement therapy Non-hormonal prescription medicines Herbal remedies and complementary therapies Lifestyle changes
Sciatica (herniated disc)	Medications Manipulation and massage Injections Surgery

account of their preferences. Patients are often ill-informed about treatment options and risks; doctors tend to underestimate patients' desire for information and they are poor at predicting patients' preferences. Wennberg, who has carried out extensive research into the practice variation phenomenon, has concluded that the answer is to change the way treatment decisions are made, replacing delegated decision-making (in which the patient delegates all responsibility for choosing treatments to the doctor) with shared decision-making. He argues that this could be achieved by changing the ethical and legal requirement of informed consent into a more active standard of informed patient choice (Wennberg 2010).

Sharing expertise

Shared decision-making takes as its starting point the notion that two types of expertise are involved in selecting treatments. The doctor is, or should be, well informed about diagnostic techniques, the causes of disease, prognosis, treatment options, and preventive strategies, but only the patient knows about his or her experience of illness, social circumstances, habits and behaviour, attitudes to risk, values and preferences. Both types of knowledge are needed to manage illness successfully, so both parties should be prepared to share information and take decisions jointly. Shared information is an essential prerequisite, but the process also depends on a commitment from both parties to engage in a negotiated decision-making process (Charles et al. 1999). The clinician must provide the patient with information about diagnosis, prognosis and treatment options, including outcome probabilities, and the patient must be prepared to discuss their values and preferences. The clinician must acknowledge the legitimacy of the patient's preferences and the patient has to accept shared responsibility for the treatment decision.

Shared decision-making draws on psychological theories about how people react to complex choices, and on evidence-based medicine, with a commitment to the application of research knowledge on the effectiveness of treatments (Mulley 2009). It explicitly recognizes the values-based nature of clinical decision-making and people's need for information and support when faced with difficult choices (Reyna 2008). So this more personalized approach aims to inform patients about the effectiveness and uncertainties inherent in treatment options for their condition, while taking account of their preferences.

In many situations there are considerable uncertainties about the likely treatment outcomes, either because these have not been sufficiently well researched or because it is not known how the patient will respond to treatment. Summarizing what is and is not known about treatment outcomes, especially when the evidence is conflicting or incomplete, is a challenging task for most clinicians, especially when faced with the conflicting pressures of a busy clinic. It requires excellent communication skills and effective educational resources, including the use of information and decision support tools for patients.

Clinician–patient relationships

The relationship between doctors and patients, and to a lesser extent between nurses or other health professionals and patients, has been of great interest to social scientists for some considerable time. As early as 1956 Szasz and Hollender set out three basic models of the doctor–patient relationship:

1 **Activity-passivity**: the patient is an entirely passive recipient of the doctor's actions.
2 **Guidance-cooperation**: an imbalance of power in which the patient is expected to cooperate in whatever action the doctor deems appropriate.
3 **Mutual participation**: a partnership in which the doctor helps the patient to help him or herself (Szasz and Hollender 1956).

The first of these is common in emergency situations when the doctor has to act quickly and there is no opportunity to consult or involve the patient. The second model, traditional paternalism, still underlies much medical practice, while the third, mutual participation, is what many clinicians are aiming to achieve; for example, in the management of chronic diseases such as diabetes.

Friedson argued that these three models were incomplete because they ignored the possibility that the patient could assume a dominant role (Friedson 1970). While this may have seemed inconceivable in 1956, nowadays there is evidence to show that clinical decisions are quite often influenced by patients' demands and expectations. For example, general practitioners often feel under pressure from parents of young children to prescribe antibiotics for minor self-limiting conditions when these are not clinically necessary (Kumar et al. 2003; Rose et al. 2006). In the past GPs bowed to this pressure because it was often the easiest thing to do, but nowadays most recognize that they need to develop strategies to help them resist the demand for unnecessary and potentially harmful treatments.

Later, Emanuel and Emanuel outlined four models to describe the increasingly complex interactions between doctors and patients – paternalistic, informative, interpretive, and deliberative (Emanuel and Emanuel 1992) (Table 4.2).

The Emanuels argued that each of the models could be appropriate in particular circumstances, but the deliberative model was the ideal, because it incorporates the idea that the clinician should help patients to reflect on their values and preferences before deciding on a course of action.

Shared decision-making and health reform

The 1990s saw an explosion of academic interest in shared decision-making and numerous papers were published elaborating on the concept. Since then, various authors have produced expanded and refined definitions that differ in various respects but generally agree on the main elements (Makoul and Clayman 2006). Many of these researchers went on to evaluate various strategies for implementing shared decision-making. A 2009 survey found a total of 27 systematic and high-quality narrative reviews that evaluated various

Table 4.2 Four models of the physician–patient relationship

	Paternalistic	Informative	Interpretive	Deliberative
Patient values	Objective and shared by physician and patient	Defined, fixed, and known to the patient	Inchoate and conflicting, requiring elucidation	Open to development and revision through moral discussion
Physician's obligation	Promoting the patient's well-being independent of the patient's current preferences	Providing relevant factual information and implementing patient's selected intervention	Elucidating and interpreting relevant patient values, as well as informing the patient and implementing the patient's selected intervention	Articulating and persuading the patient of the most admirable values, as well as informing the patient and implementing the patient's selected intervention
Conception of patient's autonomy	Assenting to objective values	Choice of, and control over, medical care	Self-understanding relevant to medical care	Moral self-development relevant to medical care
Conception of physician's role	Guardian	Competent technical expert	Counsellor or advisor	Friend or teacher

Source: Adapted from Emanuel and Emanuel (1992) with permission from the American Medical Association

initiatives designed to involve patients in making treatment choices (Picker Institute Europe 2010).

Encouraged by the relatively strong evidence base, policy-makers began to promote the idea that patients should be actively engaged in decisions about their care. For example, the NHS Constitution made the following commitments to patients in England:

- You have the right to make choices about your NHS care and to information to support these choices.
- You have the right to be involved in discussions and decisions about your healthcare, and to be given information to enable you to do this.
- You have the right to be given information about your proposed treatment in advance, including any significant risks and any alternative treatments which may be available, and the risks involved in doing nothing (Department of Health 2009).

In 2010, both the US and UK governments incorporated shared decision-making into their plans for health reform (Secretary of State for Health 2010; Senate and House of Representatives 2010). Efforts to introduce shared decision-making into mainstream clinical practice were launched by official bodies in England (Elwyn et al. 2010), in Scotland (Scottish Government 2010), in the USA (Medicare Payment Advisory Commission 2010) and in Canada (Chow et al. 2009).

Expectations of involvement

The traditional model of decision-making assumed that doctors and patients shared the same goals; that only the doctor was sufficiently informed and experienced to decide what should be done; and that patient involvement should be confined to giving or withholding consent to treatment. However, this paternalistic approach now seems seriously outdated. Nowadays many patients expect to play an active role in their own healthcare. This includes understanding the causes of their illness or disability, being informed about the prognosis and treatment options, having a say in decisions about how to treat their condition, and doing all they can to promote their recovery. While not everyone wants an active role, the majority do (Flynn et al. 2006). Surveys have found that about three-quarters of all patients expect clinicians to take account of their preferences and want to have a say in treatment decisions (Coulter and Magee 2003). The desire for participation has been found to vary according to age, educational status and disease severity, but most people in all sub-groups of the population want to feel informed and involved.

Clinicians often underestimate patients' desire for involvement and assume the role of decision-maker without checking what patients want. Patients need information about the options they face before they can decide whether to participate in the choice of treatment or leave it up to the doctor. If the doctor does not provide this information, it is very hard for the patient to express his or her preferences. The only reliable way to find out people's preferred role in treatment decision-making is to ask them, but their responses are likely to be influenced by their previous experience. Many people assume a passive role because they have never been encouraged to participate.

People's preferences may change during the course of a disease episode and their views may vary according to the severity of their condition. Patients with minor, non-life-threatening illnesses are more likely to want to be involved in selecting treatments than those with more serious conditions. For example, an Australian population survey found that more than 90 per cent expected to play an active role in decisions about diagnostic tests or treatments (Davey et al. 2002), whereas in a British survey of cancer patients only 48 per cent of those with breast cancer and only 22 per cent of those with colorectal cancer said they wanted to be involved (Beaver et al. 1999).

There are also cultural differences. A population survey carried out in eight European countries found significant variations in response to a question about who should take the lead in making treatment choices (Coulter and Magee 2003). While 91 per cent of respondents from Switzerland, 87 per cent of those from Germany and 74 per cent of those from the UK felt the patient should have a role in treatment decisions, either sharing responsibility for decision-making with the doctor or being the primary decision-maker, the proportion of Polish patients who felt the same way was only 59 per cent and in Spain it was only 44 per cent.

Younger and better educated people are more likely to say they want to play an active role, but age on its own is not a reliable predictor of people's preferences (Kennelly and Bowling 2001; O'Connor et al. 2003). Older people are particularly likely to suffer from the presumption that they are incapable of taking decisions or unwilling to face choices about their medical care. Care of patients at the end of life is a case in point. National guidance requires that do-not-rescuscitate orders should not be applied without first discussing the issue with patients and/or their relatives, yet there is evidence that this frequently does not happen (Bowling and Ebrahim 2001).

Lack of involvement in decisions

Despite an expectation of involvement on the part of many patients, the evidence suggests that patients are not usually encouraged to share their beliefs, experiences and expectations. Doctors often focus more on the disease than the person and do not explore patients' values and preferences (Corke et al. 2005). A review of 134 observational studies of communication between patients and practitioners about medicine-taking found that most patients were happy to discuss their concerns, but health professionals did not encourage them to do so (Stevenson et al. 2004). Doctors tended to dominate discussion in the consultation and patients tended to take a passive role. Patients often failed to disclose to clinicians that they had not taken the medicines as recommended, and when providing information, doctors rarely assessed patients' understanding of it, despite an awareness of the importance of doing so. In short, there was scant evidence of genuine two-way communication and often relevant information was not shared.

The national surveys of NHS patients in England provide further evidence that large numbers of patients are disappointed about the lack of opportunity to have a say in clinical decisions (Care Quality Commission 2010). When asked whether they had been sufficiently involved in decisions about their care, only half of hospital inpatients said they were involved as much as they wanted to be and the trend remained virtually static between 2002 and 2008, suggesting a large unmet demand for greater involvement (Figure 4.1).

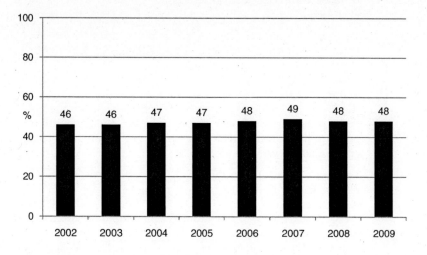

Source: NHS national inpatient surveys, Care Quality Commission

Figure 4.1 Proportion of inpatients who wanted more involvement in treatment decisions

Informed consent

Informed consent is the term traditionally used to describe the patient's role in decision-making. The doctrine of informed consent derives from the ethical principle of autonomy (ensuring that patients' beliefs and preferences are respected and they are supported in making choices), but medical ethics also requires doctors to take account of beneficence (doing good and avoiding harm) and justice (treating all patients equally). In its guidance on informed consent the UK General Medical Council (GMC) placed great stress on the autonomy principle:

> Whatever the context in which medical decisions are made, you must work in partnership with your patients to ensure good care. In so doing, you must listen to patients and respect their views about their health; discuss with patients what their diagnosis, prognosis, treatment and care involve; share with patients the information they want or need in order to make decisions; maximise patients' opportunities, and their ability, to make decisions for themselves; respect patients' decisions.
>
> (General Medical Council 2008: 6)

Patients cannot express informed preferences unless they have appropriate information, including an understanding of their condition and the likely outcomes with and without treatment. There is a professional and moral consensus about the clinical duty to obtain informed consent, but a legal requirement to do so extends only to surgical procedures and entry into clinical trials. In surgical practice, obtaining informed consent has often been viewed as a passive activity where the goal is to obtain the patient's signature to indicate acquiescence to a treatment that the doctor has selected. Doctors have tended to talk about 'consenting the patient', using it as a transitive verb to denote something that is done *to* the patient instead of *with* them, a passive rather than an active, participative decision-making process.

However, this is beginning to change as a result of growing interest in new models of clinician–patient interaction that involve a shift away from the essentially passive notion of informed consent to a more active and participative model of informed patient choice or shared decision-making. Robert Veatch has argued that informed consent has had its day:

> It remains, however, a relic of modern medicine, a minimal movement in the direction of recognizing the role of the active, responsible patient in his or her own medical decisions. If patients are ever to become active decision makers controlling their own health and healing based on their own beliefs and values, we will have to do better.
>
> (Veatch 2009: 102)

Seeking to improve practice in informed consent, the General Medical Council has detailed the information that patients may want to know, before deciding whether to consent to treatment or an investigation (General Medical Council 2008) (Figure 4.2).

In effect the General Medical Council has redefined the definition of informed consent to align it with shared decision-making. However, it is not clear that the courts would take the same view (King and Moulton 2006). New laws may be required to mandate shared decision-making. This process is beginning to happen in some US states. For example, the State of Washington passed legislation in 2007 to make it clear that shared decision-making gives greater legal protection for doctors than the standard means of obtaining informed consent (Moulton and King 2010). This may prove to be a powerful driver to improve the way medical decisions are made.

You must give patients the information they want or need about:

a) the diagnosis and prognosis
b) any uncertainties about the diagnosis or prognosis, including options for further investigations
c) options for treating or managing the condition, including the option not to treat
d) the purpose of any proposed investigation or treatment and what it will involve
e) the potential benefits, risks and burdens, and the likelihood of success, for each option; this should include information, if available, about whether the benefits or risks are affected by which organisation or doctor is chosen to provide care
f) whether a proposed investigation or treatment is part of a research programme or is an innovative treatment designed specifically for their benefit
g) the people who will be mainly responsible for and involved in their care, what their roles are, and to what extent students may be involved
h) their right to refuse to take part in teaching or research
i) their right to seek a second opinion
j) any bills they will have to pay
k) any conflicts of interest that you, or your organisation, may have
l) any treatments that you believe have greater potential benefit for the patient than those you or your organisation can offer.

Source: General Medical Council (2008)

Figure 4.2 GMC guidance on informed consent

Patient decision aids

Patient decision aids have been developed to support shared decision-making. These take a variety of forms including web applications, videos/DVDs, computer programs, leaflets and structured counselling. They differ from standard information packages in that they are designed to:

- provide facts about the disease or condition, treatment options and the benefits, harms and uncertainties of each of these
- outline the outcome probabilities tailored to an individual's risk factors
- help clarify patients' evaluations of the outcomes that matter most to them
- guide patients in the steps of decision-making and communicating their preferences.

Decision aids are evidence-based tools designed to facilitate the process of making informed values-based choices about disease management and treatment options, prevention or screening. They are intended to supplement rather than replace patient–clinician interaction. The content is based on reviews of clinical research and studies of patients' information needs. They do not tell people what they should do. Instead they aim to help patients clarify their values and preferences and weigh up the potential benefits and harms of alternative courses of action.

Decision aids take a variety of forms, but most include the following characteristics (Elwyn et al. 2009):

- They explicitly recognize patients' role in the clinical decision-making process.
- They describe clinical procedures and patients' experience of undergoing these.
- They identify key decision points along a care pathway where the patient's views are important.
- They list the treatment options and summarize the likely outcomes in such a way as to enable comparison.
- They provide information about the strength of the research evidence and any uncertainties.
- They present risks and probabilities in a clear, quantified way.
- They provide support for clarifying and expressing values.
- They avoid biased presentation and over-promotion of particular options.
- They include information about sources of research evidence and citations.
- They include information about authorship and funding sources.

Decision aids can be used in a wide variety of clinical situations, including the following:

- Symptom management and triage to the most appropriate level of care, including self-care (e.g. sore throat, diarrhoea, minor head injury).
- Conditions or health risks where there is more than one treatment or screening option, requiring careful weighing of benefits and harms of each, including the option of no treatment (e.g. menstrual disorders, lower urinary tract symptoms, prostate cancer screening).
- Chronic condition management to determine the patient's goals and behaviour change priorities (e.g. managing diabetes, asthma, hypertension, or end-of-life care).

Use of evidence-based decision aids for patients has been shown to lead to improvements in knowledge, better understanding of treatment options and more accurate perception of risks (O'Connor et al. 2009). Decision aids help to increase patient involvement in decision-making and increase patients' confidence in the process. They also produce a better match between patients' preferences and the treatments chosen, leading to increased satisfaction. There is no evidence that they make patients more anxious.

One of the encouraging aspects of using decision aids to inform and engage patients is that in some cases this can improve cost-effectiveness. Patients who are fully informed about the pros and cons of treatments often opt for the least invasive, and least costly option. For example, a study to evaluate the use of decision support for women referred to gynaecology outpatients because of excessive menstrual bleeding found that those that received the intervention (a video and booklet explaining the treatment options and likely outcomes plus a structured interview with a nurse to help them clarify their preferences) led to a significant reduction in the proportion opting for hysterectomy and considerably lower treatment costs (Kennedy et al. 2002). Studies have found similar reductions in the use of other elective surgical procedures when patients are given clear information and effective decision support (O'Connor et al. 2009).

Many decision aids are quite sophisticated, including videos, computerized risk calculation tools and printed booklets. Some experts have argued that the best can be the enemy of the good when it comes to designing decision aids. A good quality information leaflet and a values clarification exercise may be sufficient, especially if it is coupled with the chance to talk through the decision with a knowledgeable but neutral person. It is, however, very important to ensure that the materials conform to agreed standards of accuracy and design (Elwyn et al. 2009).

While use of decision aids has been slow to filter into mainstream clinical practice, the situation is beginning to change as a consequence of the promotion and funding of demonstration sites in the USA, the UK and elsewhere, funded by organizations such as the Foundation for Informed Medical Decision Making in Boston and the Health Foundation in London. A commitment in President Obama's health reform bill, which was signed into law in March 2010, is likely to hasten the adoption of this approach. The intention is to create a programme to facilitate shared decision-making, to develop, test and certify patient decision aids, and to create shared decision-making resource centres and demonstration projects to study the effects of giving patients a more powerful role in medical decision-making (Senate and House of Representatives 2010). Similar efforts are under way in the UK and other European countries, perhaps presaging a major culture change in respect of attitudes to patient engagement.

Risk communication

Risk communication involves providing factual information about outcome probabilities, helping people to weigh up the balance of likely benefits and harms and confront uncertainties. It is a key component of the shared decision-making process, but it requires considerable knowledge and skill to do it effectively. Many people, including many doctors, find understanding statistics and probabilities quite difficult. Communicating these clearly can be quite a challenge for clinicians. Even basic mathematical concepts like percentages can be confusing to some people.

Gigerenzer and his colleagues have drawn attention to the widespread problem of statistical illiteracy in healthcare that affects doctors, patients, journalists and politicians alike (Gigerenzer et al. 2008). They point to examples such as the 1995 contraceptive pill scare that caused a rise in unwanted pregnancies and abortions largely due to the way the results were presented. People were alarmed by reports that taking low-dose hormonal contraceptives could lead to a twofold increase in relative risk of thrombosis. In fact the absolute (population-based) risk increase was only 1 in 7,000, a much less alarming figure. Talking about the *relative* risk without providing information about the underlying occurrence in the population (*absolute* risk) can be very misleading. This type of confusion in how to interpret research findings can also befuddle doctors. For example, only 79 per cent of gynaecologists were able to accurately interpret figures on the likelihood that a woman who tests positive in mammography screening actually has breast cancer (Gigerenzer et al. 2008). The situation is not helped by the fact that research papers in medical journals often fail to report the underlying absolute risks (Gigerenzer et al. 2010).

Given these difficulties, it is clear that both doctors and patients need help with communicating and understanding risk. Fortunately, how best to communicate risk has been fairly well studied (Bunge et al. 2010; Thomson et al. 2005). While there is no perfect solution, it is generally agreed that the guidelines outlined in Table 4.3 can aid understanding.

Well-designed decision aids usually incorporate these ways of presenting risk, saving time for the clinician and removing the need to remember the detailed results of clinical trials.

Support for participation

The provision of information and decision aids can be helpful for patients, but they may need additional support if they are to play an active role in consultations. Promising interventions include health coaches who help patients deliberate about their options and encourage them to raise concerns and express their preferences, question cards that suggest appropriate questions to ask the doctor, and provision of summaries or audiotapes of the main points discussed for the patient to review after the consultation.

Researchers at the Ottawa Hospital Research Institute at the University of Ottawa in Canada have developed a framework for decision support (O'Connor and Jacobsen 2007). This outlines ways in which people can be helped to deal with difficult medical decisions. Based on theories from psychology and

Table 4.3 Communicating risk

Guidance	Examples
Explain uncertainty	No diagnostic test is completely accurate, explain the likelihood of false positive and false negative results: 'Of 1,000 women who do not have mammography, four will die of breast cancer in the next 10 years, whereas out of 1,000 who do have mammography, three will die'
Do not rely on words alone – quantify where possible	'More women had a blood clot in their leg or lungs when taking drug X (an additional 5 in 1,000 due to the drug)'
Use event rates (natural frequencies) not percentages or relative risks	'Of 100 people like you, five will have a stroke in the next year'
Use specific time frames	'The probability that a 50-year-old British woman will die of colon cancer in the next 10 years is 2 in 1,000'
Constant denominators are better than constant numerators	'1 out of 1,000; 14 out of 1,000'; this is better than '1 in 100, 1 in 20'
Use both positive and negative framing where possible	'Two years after external beam radiotherapy for prostate cancer, about 3 to 5 men out of 100 wear pads to help deal with wetness, and a similar number have problems urinating and controlling the flow of urine. About 94 to 97 men out of 100 do not have these problems'
Use simple graphics such as bar charts	People understand bar charts better than more complex graphics; pie charts are not as well understood
Give individually tailored probabilities adjusted for baseline risk where possible	Computerized predictive risk scores can be helpful to illustrate the likelihood that an individual will experience a particular outcome

decision analysis, it recognizes that many healthcare decisions involve weighing up options that have both desirable and undesirable outcomes when the desirable outcomes occur partly with one option and partly with another. This situation, when no option is self-evidently best, is known as a 'choice dilemma' or 'conflicted decision'. When faced with these difficult decisions people feel unsure about what to do and they may worry about the consequences of whatever they might decide, leading them to dither or delay and sometimes causing them considerable distress.

Effective counselling, also known as decision coaching, can help by clarifying the choices, addressing knowledge deficits, helping people to consider their personal values, and by providing structured guidance in the steps of decision-making. A good decision is one that is informed and values-based; in other words, it is consistent with people's informed preferences. Rather than leaping to a decision without considering the consequences, health coaches help patients think through the options step by step. They use listening skills, open and closed questions, and reflective feedback, carefully tailored to people's individual needs and drawing on motivational interviewing techniques (Rollnick et al. 2010). This type of support can help patients determine which option is best for them, sometimes leading to decisions that are very different from those that might have been made for them by doctors without their active participation (Kennedy et al. 2002).

Encouraging patients to prepare relevant questions prior to consultation leads to more question-asking, but this does not always lead to improvements in their knowledge, perhaps because not all clinicians are good communicators. For example, a systematic review identified 33 randomized controlled trials involving 8,244 patients from six countries, mainly the USA, in a range of clinical settings (Kinnersley et al. 2009). These studies evaluated question prompts and coaching usually delivered in the waiting room immediately before the consultation for patients with a variety of health problems. The interventions led to small increases in question-asking and some improvements in patient satisfaction, but no other clear benefits. Another review of interventions designed to encourage older people to play a more active role in consultations found very similar results (Wetzels et al. 2008).

It is known that patients often cannot remember all the details of what they are told in consultations. This is especially true when they receive bad news, such as diagnosis of a serious condition. It is hard to take everything in when you have been told you have a serious condition. Initial reactions of fear and anxiety can prevent you absorbing any further information. In these situations some patients find it helpful to have a record of the main points to review when they get home. This can act as a personal reminder, to inform their families or friends, or even to replay to their general practitioners for later discussion (Scott et al. 2003). In a hospital in California, trained facilitators attend breast cancer consultations to take notes and then use these in later discussions with patients to clarify what they were told by the specialist and to think through their attitudes to the treatment options (Belkora et al. 2008).

Advance care plans

Advance care plans, also called advance directives, living wills, advance decisions, or advance statements, are documents that allow people to specify what should happen if they lose mental capacity in the future. These often have legal force although there are some limitations: for example, they cannot be used to request euthanasia or to force doctors to act against their professional judgement, nor to nominate someone else to make decisions on your behalf – for that it is necessary to apply for power of attorney. Nevertheless, they do provide a way for people to exert some control over what happens to them when they are terminally ill.

While mostly thought of as useful for people with terminal illness, advance care plans can also be used by people who have a serious mental illness to specify which treatments they wish to avoid during a psychotic episode (Amering et al. 2005). They can be used to refuse some or all forms of medical treatment, but not to request specific treatments. For example, people who are terminally ill may wish to refuse consent in advance for cardiopulmonary resuscitation, mechanical ventilation, artificial nutrition or antibiotics.

In England the Medical Capacity Act of 2005 specified that to be valid advance care plans must:

- be made by a person who is 18 or over and has the capacity to make it
- specify the treatment to be refused
- specify the circumstances in which this refusal would apply
- not have been made under the influence or harassment of anyone else
- not have been modified verbally or in writing since it was made (Department of Constitutional Affairs 2007).

Advance decisions to refuse life-sustaining treatment (do-not-resuscitate orders), must be in writing, be signed and witnessed, and must include an express statement that the decision stands 'even if life is at risk'. While some older people welcome the opportunity to have more control over what happens to them at the end of life, others find it distressing to think about their preferences in advance (Seymour et al. 2004). Most will need sensitive help from professional staff to participate in an advance care planning process (Davison and Simpson 2006). Ideally they should have an opportunity to consider alternative future scenarios based on careful descriptions of the likely effects of intervention. This can be facilitated by the use of video clips.

Studies of elderly patients faced with a choice of life-prolonging care involving invasive procedures, limited or basic care involving less invasive treatment, or comfort care only have found that video clips help them understand and focus on the experience of patients and their families when undergoing the different forms of care (Deep et al. 2010). Randomized trials comparing verbal descriptions alone and verbal descriptions with videos have shown that those viewing the videos are much more likely to opt for less invasive forms of treatment when preparing a care plan (El-Jawahri et al. 2010; Volandes et al. 2009). Videos such as these can be especially useful for helping low literacy patients understand their options and express their preferences and these patients value the opportunity to view them (Volandes et al. 2008b; Volandes et al. 2008a).

In practice, advance care plans can be difficult to apply unless the patient's wishes are completely clear, the circumstances of their mental incapacity were accurately foreseen, and their next of kin fully accept these (Bonner et al. 2009). Studies in the USA have suggested that, at least until recently, many patients did not have an opportunity to participate in effective advance planning for terminal care (Kass-Bartelmes and Hughes 2003). Less than 50 per cent had an advance care plan in their medical record and, of those that did, few of their doctors were aware of its existence, so their wishes were ignored. There is very little robust evidence on the impact of using advance care plans in mental health, although one study suggested they may help to reduce hospital admissions and compulsory treatment (Campbell and Kisely 2009).

Improving decision quality

The last 20 years or so have seen concerted efforts to encourage clinicians to adopt an evidence-based approach when treating patients. Evidence of widespread variations in clinical practice demonstrates the fact that practice is often far from evidence based at present (Mulley 2010; Wennberg 2010). Governments, health authorities, charities and commercial organizations have expended considerable sums on funding clinical trials and systematic reviews designed to improve understanding of what works in medical care and what does not. These have given rise to clinical guidelines setting out treatment recommendations based on the results of the trials. This effort has played a key role in improving the quality and effectiveness of healthcare, but it has become apparent that guidelines cannot be applied slavishly in all instances, since individual patients respond differently and often have different preferences and attitudes to risk. This recognition has contributed to the new emphasis on patient involvement and personalization, with a focus on promoting a more equal, participative approach to decision-making.

There are three main reasons why involving patients in a shared decision-making process is now seen as the best way to select treatments when there is more than one option:

1 a belief that giving patients a say in what happens to them is 'the right thing to do' and accords with the ethical principle of autonomy
2 an improvement on current informed consent procedures
3 a means of ensuring that patients receive the tests and procedures they want and need, no more and no less.

Yet, as we have seen, clinicians have been slow to relinquish their traditional role as the sole decision-maker and many patients are frustrated by an inability to influence what happens to them. Sometimes, treatment choices are presented to patients, but in a biased manner, with clinicians effectively downplaying all options other than the ones they favour.

Building on the dictum that what gets measured is what matters, some have argued that what is needed is a way of measuring the quality of the decision-making process to focus minds on how to encourage patient engagement instead of blocking it (Sepucha et al. 2004). Decision quality refers to the extent to which treatment or management decisions reflect the considered preferences of well-informed patients and are implemented. The key issues that should be measured are:

- How informed was the patient about the key things a person should know (benefits, harms or uncertainties) before embarking on a particular treatment, screening or care management programme?
- To what extent was the decision personalized to reflect the patient's goals? Did the treatment selected match their preferences?
- Did the clinician give serious attention to informing and involving the patient in the decision process? (Sepucha et al. 2008)

Overcoming the barriers

Despite the policy commitment to promote patient engagement in managing care, and evidence of benefit, widespread implementation of innovations such as those described in this chapter has yet to occur. The resistance comes from professionals in the main, not patients. Barriers include lack of awareness, lack of incentives, lack of knowledge and skills, concerns about time and resource pressures, and negative attitudes among some clinicians because of possible loss of power, loss of face or loss of income (Coulter 2010). Shared decision-making involves a reorientation from traditional paternalistic models of practice towards new forms of thinking about clinician–patient relations. This is not easy for practitioners who are wedded to a clinician-centred model of decision-making. Like any proposed change in healthcare delivery, professionals need to be convinced that the advantages to patients outweigh the perceived disadvantages of adapting their traditional routines.

Overcoming the many barriers to change necessitates paying attention to incentives for professionals, patients and managers to make the required adaptations to the clinical context in which they are working. Time pressures are frequently cited as a reason for not involving patients more actively (Legare et al. 2008). Other barriers include in-built inertia that inhibits changes to regular routines and care pathways, and the prevailing medical culture which still tends towards paternalism. Formal training can help to overcome resistance (Lewin et al. 2001). This involves teaching professionals to respect patients' autonomy, a skill that can be taught but must not be taken for granted.

Changing the way healthcare is delivered is a complex process. The Normalisation Process Model, which focuses attention on how complex interventions become routinely embedded in practice, provides a structure for understanding the relationships between a complex intervention such as shared decision-making and the context in which it is implemented, paying attention to the process of implementation, the required skill set, integration into existing routines, and patterns of interpersonal behaviour (Elwyn et al. 2008). In Figure 4.3 it is applied to the implementation of patient decision support technologies (DST).

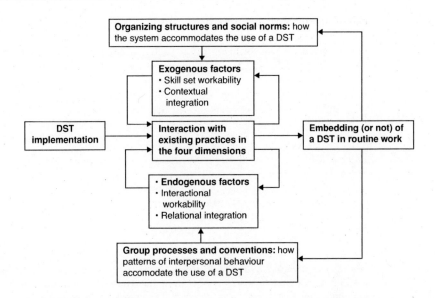

Source: Elwyn et al. (2008)

Figure 4.3 Normalization process model and patient decision support

As well as considering the interaction between patient and professional, the model points to the need to take account of professional and organizational norms that are typically oriented to clinician-led decision-making instead of preference-sensitive decision-making by patients. It may be necessary to realign incentives so that clinicians are actively encouraged to involve patients in decisions and to monitor their accomplishment of the task. Training would be provided and patient engagement would be incorporated into clinical guidelines, using feedback from patients to check progress. Health professionals and managers would require evidence of the use of decision aids in performance targets. Relevant metrics might include the percentage of patients who report having had the opportunity to make informed decisions, or disease-specific measures of decision quality such as those described above. Such metrics could be incorporated into accreditation and reimbursement strategies.

Summary

Shared decision-making is a process in which patients are involved as active partners with clinicians in clarifying acceptable medical options and in choosing a preferred course of clinical care. It represents a step change from the traditional doctor–patient relationship in which only the doctor's expertise was recognized and the patient's role was simply to follow the doctor's orders. As well as providing facts and figures to help the patient make an informed choice, the clinician should help the patient consider their options and the likely outcomes and engage them in a process of deliberation to determine their preferred course of action. Effective risk communication, the use of evidence-based patient decision aids and decision coaching can help with this process. Despite evidence of benefit, these initiatives to empower patients have been slow to filter into mainstream clinical practice.

References

Amering, M., Stastny, P. and Hopper, K. (2005) Psychiatric advance directives: qualitative study of informed deliberations by mental health service users, *British Journal of Psychiatry*, 186: 247–52.

Beaver, K., Bogg, J. and Luker, K. A. (1999) Decision-making role preferences and information needs: a comparison of colorectal and breast cancer, *Health Expectations*, 2: 266–76.

Belkora, J.K., Loth, M.K., Chen, D.F., Chen, J.Y., Volz, S. and Esserman, L.J. (2008) Monitoring the implementation of Consultation Planning, Recording, and Summarizing in a breast care center, *Patient Education and Counseling*, 73(3): 536–43.

Bonner, S., Tremlett, M. and Bell, D. (2009) Are advance directives legally binding or simply the starting point for discussion on patients' best interests?, *British Medical Journal*, 339: b4667.

Bowling, A. and Ebrahim, S. (2001) Measuring patients' preferences for treatment and perceptions of risk, *Quality in Health Care*, 10(suppl. 1): i12–18.

Bunge, M., Muhlhauser, I. and Steckelberg. A. (2010) What constitutes evidence-based patient information? Overview of discussed criteria, *Patient Education and Counseling*, 78: 316–28.

Campbell, L.A. and Kisely, S.R. (2009) Advance treatment directives for people with severe mental illness, *Cochrane Database System Review*, 1: CD005963.

Care Quality Commission (2010) *Inpatient Survey 2009*. Newcastle: Care Quality Commission.

Charles, C., Gafni, A. and Whelan, T. (1999) Decision-making in the physician-patient encounter: revisiting the shared treatment decision-making model, *Social Science and Medicine*, 49(5): 651–61.

Chow, S., Teare, G. and Basky, G. (2009) *Shared Decision Making: Helping the System and Patients Make Quality Health Care Decisions*. Saskatoon: Health Quality Council.

Collins, E.D., Moore, C.P., Clay, K.F., Kearing, S.A., O'Connor, A.M., Llewellyn-Thomas, H.A., Barth, R.J., Jr. and Sepucha, K.R. (2009) Can women with early-stage breast cancer make an informed decision for mastectomy?, *Journal of Clinical Oncology*, 27(4): 519–25.

Corke, C.F., Stow, P.J., Green, D.T., Agar, J.W. and Henry, M.J. (2005) How doctors discuss major interventions with high risk patients: an observational study, *British Medical Journal*, 330: 182–84.

Coulter, A. (2010) *Implementing Shared Decision Making in the UK*. London: Health Foundation.

Coulter, A. and Magee, H. (2003) *The European Patient of the Future*. Maidenhead: Open University Press.

Davey, H.M., Barratt, A.L., Davey, E., Butow, P.N., Redman, S., Houssami, N. and Salkeld, G.P. (2002) Medical tests: women's reported and preferred decision-making roles and preferences for information on benefits, side-effects and false results, *Health Expectations*, 5(4): 330–40.

Davison, S.N. and Simpson, C. (2006) Hope and advance care planning in patients with end stage renal disease: qualitative interview study, *British Medical Journal*, 333(7574): 886.

Deep, K.S., Hunter, A., Murphy, K. and Volandes, A. (2010) 'It helps me see with my heart': how video informs patients' rationale for decisions about future care in advanced dementia, *Patient Education and Counseling*, 81(2): 229–34.

Department of Constitutional Affairs (2007) *Mental Capacity Act 2005: Code of Practice*. London: The Stationery Office.

Department of Health (2009) *The NHS Constitution*. London: Department of Health.

El-Jawahri, A., Podgurski, L.M., Eichler, A.F., Plotkin, S.R., Temel, J.S., Mitchell, S.L., Chang, Y., Barry, M.J. and Volandes, A.E. (2010) Use of video to facilitate end-of-life discussions with patients with cancer: a randomized controlled trial, *Journal of Clinical Oncology*, 28(2): 305–10.

Elwyn, G., Laitner, S., Coulter, A., Walker, E., Watson, P. and Thomson, R. (2010) Implementing shared decision making in the NHS, *British Medical Journal*, 341: c5146.

Elwyn, G., Legare, F., Weijden, T., Edwards, A. and May, C. (2008) Arduous implementation: does the Normalisation Process Model explain why it's so difficult to embed decision support technologies for patients in routine clinical practice, *Implementation Science*, 3: 57.

Elwyn, G., O'Connor, A.M., Bennett, C., Newcombe, R.G., Politi, M., Durand, M.A., Drake, E., Joseph-Williams, N., Khangura, S., Saarimaki, A., Sivell, S., Stiel, M., Bernstein, S.J., Col, N., Coulter, A., Eden, K., Harter, M., Rovner, M.H., Moumjid, N., Stacey, D., Thomson, R., Whelan, T., van der, W.T. and Edwards, A. (2009) Assessing the quality of decision support technologies using the International Patient Decision Aid Standards instrument (IPDASi), *PLoS ONE*, 4(3): e4705.

Emanuel, E.J. and Emanuel, L.L. (1992) Four models of the physician-patient relationship, *Journal of the American Association*, 267(16): 2221–26.

Fagerlin, A., Sepucha, K.R., Couper, M.P., Levin, C.A., Singer, E. and Zikmund-Fisher, B.J. (2010) Patients' knowledge about 9 common health conditions: The DECISIONS Survey, *Medical Decision Making*, 30(5 suppl): 35S–52S.

Flynn, K.E., Smith, M.A. and Vanness, D. (2006) A typology of preferences for participation in healthcare decision making, *Social Science and Medicine*, 63(5): 1158–69.

Friedson, E. (1970) *The Profession of Medicine*. New York: Dodd Mead & Co.

General Medical Council (2008) *Consent: Patients and Doctors Making Decisions Together*. London: GMC.

Gigerenzer, G., Gaissmaier, W., Kurz-Milcke, E., Schwartz, L.M. and Woloshin, S. (2008) Helping doctors and patients make sense of health statistics, *Psychological Science in the Public Interest*, 8(2): 53–96.

Gigerenzer, G., Wegwarth, O. and Feufel, M. (2010) Misleading communication of risk, *British Medical Journal*, 341: c4830.

Grol, R., Wensing, M., Mainz, J., Jung, H.P., Ferreira, P., Hearnshaw, H., Hjortdahl, P., Olesen, F., Reis, S., Ribacke, M. and Szecsenyi, J. (2000) Patients in Europe evaluate general practice care: an international comparison, *British Journal of General Practice*, 50(460): 882–87.

Kass-Bartelmes, B.L. and Hughes, R. (2003) Advance care planning: preferences for care at the end of life, *Research in Action*, 12. Available online at www.ahrq.gov/research/endliferia/endria.htm; accessed 17 May 2011.

Kennedy, A.D., Sculpher, M.J., Coulter, A., Dwyer, N., Rees, M., Abrams, K.R., Horsley, S., Cowley, D., Kidson, C., Kirwin, C., Naish, C. and Stirrat, G. (2002) Effects of decision aids for menorrhagia on treatment choices, health outcomes, and costs: a randomized controlled trial, *Journal of the American Association*, 288(21): 2701–8.

Kennelly, C. and Bowling, A. (2001) Suffering in deference: a focus group study of older cardiac patients' preferences for treatment and perceptions of risk, *Quality in Health Care*, 10(Suppl. 1): i23–i28.

King, J.S. and Moulton, B. (2006) Rethinking informed consent: the case for shared medical decision-making, *American Journal of Law and Medicine*, 32: 429–501.

Kinnersley, P., Edwards, A., Hood, K., Cadbury, N., Ryan, R., Prout, H., Owen, D., MacBeth, F., Butow, P. and Butler, C. (2009) Interventions before consultations before helping patients address their information needs, *Cochrane Database of Systematic Review* (Online), vol. 1.

Kumar, S., Little, P. and Britten, N. (2003) Why do general practitioners prescribe antibiotics for sore throat? Grounded theory interview study, *British Medical Journal*, 326: 138–43.

Legare, F., Ratte, S., Gravel, K. and Graham, I.D. (2008) Barriers and facilitators to implementing shared decision-making in clinical practice: update of a systematic review of health professionals' perceptions, *Patient Education and Counseling*, 73(3): 526–35.

Lewin, S.A., Skea, Z.C., Entwistle, V., Zwarenstein, M. and Dick, J. (2001) Interventions for providers to promote a patient-centred approach in clinical consultations, *Cochrane Database Systematic Review*, 4: CD003267.

Makoul, G. and Clayman, M.L. (2006) An integrative model of shared decision making in medical encounters, *Patient Education and Counseling*, 60(3): 301–12.

Medicare Payment Advisory Commission (2010) Shared decision making and its implications for Medicare, in MedPAC (ed.) *Aligning incentives in Medicare: Report to the Congress* (pp. 191–210). Washington, DC: MedPAC.

Moulton, B. and King, J.S. (2010) Aligning ethics with medical decision-making: the quest for informed patient choice, *Journal of Law, Medicine and Ethics*, 38(1): 85–97.

Mulley, A.G. (2009) Inconvenient truths about supplier induced demand and unwarranted variation in medical practice, *British Medical Journal*, 339: b4073.

Mulley, A.G. (2010) Improving productivity in the NHS, *British Medical Journal*, 341: c3965.

O'Connor, A., Drake, E.R., Wells, G.A., Tugwell, P., Laupacis, A. and Elmslie, T. (2003) A survey of the decision-making needs of Canadians faced with complex health decisions, *Health Expectations*, 6(2): 97–109.

O'Connor, A. M. and Jacobsen, M.J. (2007) Decisional conflict: supporting people experiencing uncertainty about options affecting their health, Ottawa Hospital Research Institute, University of Ottawa.

O'Connor, A.M., Bennett, C.L., Stacey, D., Barry, M., Col, N.F., Eden, K.B., Entwistle, V.A., Fiset, V., Holmes-Rovner, M., Khangura, S., Llewellyn-Thomas, H. and Rovner, D. (2009) Decision aids for people facing health treatment or screening decisions, *Cochrane Database Systematic Review*, 3: CD001431.

O'Connor, A.M., Wennberg, J.E., Legare, F., Llewellyn-Thomas, H.A., Moulton, B.W., Sepucha, K.R., Sodano, A.G. and King, J.S. (2007) Toward the 'tipping point': decision aids and informed patient choice, *Health Aff (Millwood)*, 26(3): 716–25.

Picker Institute Europe (2010) *Invest in Engagement*. Oxford: Picker Institute Europe.

Reyna, V.F. (2008) Theories of medical decision making and health: an evidence-based approach, *Medical Decision Making*, 28(6): 829–33.

Right Care (2010) *NHS Atlas of Variation in Healthcare: Reducing Unwarranted Variation to Increase Value and Improve Quality.* London: Department of Health.

Rollnick, S., Butler, C.C., Kinnersley, P., Gregory, J. and Mash, B. (2010) Motivational interviewing, *British Medical Journal*, 340: 1242–45.

Rose, P.W., Ziebland, S., Harnden, A., Mayon-White, R. and Mant, D. (2006) Why do general practitioners prescribe antibiotics for acute infective conjunctivitis in children? Qualitative interviews with GPs and a questionnaire survey of parents and teachers, *Family Practice*, 23(2): 226–32.

Scott, J.T., Harmsen, M., Prictor, M.J., Entwistle, V.A., Sowden, A.J. and Watt, I. (2003) Recordings or summaries of consultations for people with cancer, *Cochrane Database Systematic Review*, 2: CD001539.

Scottish Government (2010) *The Healthcare Quality Strategy for NHS Scotland.* Edinburgh: Scottish Government.

Secretary of State for Health (2010) *Equity and Excellence: Liberating the NHS*, (Cmd. 7881). London: The Stationery Office.

Senate and House of Representatives (2010) *Patient Protection and Affordable Care Act*, (HR 3590). Washington, DC: US Congress.

Sepucha, K.R., Fowler, F.J., Jr. and Mulley, A.G., Jr. (2004) Policy support for patient-centered care: the need for measurable improvements in decision quality, *Health Aff. (Millwood)*, Suppl. Web Exclusives: VAR54–VAR62.

Sepucha, K.R., Levin, C.A., Uzogara, E.E., Barry, M.J., O'Connor, A.M. and Mulley, A.G. (2008) Developing instruments to measure the quality of decisions: early results for a set of symptom-driven decisions, *Patient Education and Counseling*, 73(3): 504–10.

Seymour, J., Gott, M., Bellamy, G., Ahmedzai, S.H. and Clark, D. (2004) Planning for the end of life: the views of older people about advance care statements, *Social Science and Medicine*, 59(1): 57–68.

Stevenson, F.A., Cox, K., Britten, N. and Dundar, Y. (2004) A systematic review of the research on communication between patients and health care professionals about medicines: the consequences for concordance, *Health Expectations*, 7(3): 235–45.

Szasz, T.S. and Hollender, M.H. (1956) A contribution to the philosophy of medicine: the basic models of the doctor-patient relationship, *Archives of Internal Medicine*, 97: 585–92.

Thomson, R., Edwards, A. and Grey, J. (2005) Risk communication in the clinical consultation, *Clinical Medicine*, 5(5): 465–69.

Veatch, R.M. (2009) *Patient, Heal Thyself: How the New Medicine Puts the Patient in Charge.* Oxford: Oxford University Press.

Volandes, A.E., Ariza, M., Abbo, E.D. and Paasche-Orlow, M. (2008a) Overcoming educational barriers for advance care planning in Latinos with video images, *Journal of Palliative Medicine*, 11(5): 700–6.

Volandes, A.E., Paasche-Orlow, M., Gillick, M.R., Cook, E.F., Shaykevich, S., Abbo, E.D. and Lehmann, L. (2008b) Health literacy not race predicts end-of-life care preferences, *Journal of Palliative Medicine*, 11(5): 754–62.

Volandes, A.E., Paasche-Orlow, M.K., Barry, M.J., Gillick, M.R., Minaker, K.L., Chang, Y., Cook, E.F., Abbo, E.D., El-Jawahri, A. and Mitchell, S.L. (2009) Video decision support tool for advance care planning in dementia: randomised controlled trial, *British Medical Journal*, 338: b2159.

Wennberg, J.E. (2010) *Tracking Medicine: A Researcher's Quest to Understand Health Care.* Oxford: Oxford University Press.

Wetzels, R., Harmsen, M., van Weel, C., Grol, R. and Wensing, M. (2008) Interventions for improving older patients' involvement in primary care episodes, *Cochrane Database of Systematic Review* (Online), vol. 4.

Zikmund-Fisher, B.J., Couper, M.P., Singer, E., Ubel, P.A., Ziniel, S., Fowler, F.J., Levin, C.A. and Fagerlin, A. (2010) Deficits and variations in patients' experience with making 9 common medical decisions: The DECISIONS Survey, *Medical Decision Making*, 30(Suppl. 5): 85S–95S.

Further reading

Edwards A. and Elwyn G. (2009) *Shared Decision-making in Health Care*, 2nd edn. Oxford: Oxford University Press.

Gigerenzer G. (2002) *Reckoning with Risk: Learning to Live with Uncertainty*. London: Penguin Books.

Goldacre B. (2009) *Bad Science*. London: Harper Perennial.

Katz J. (2002) *The Silent World of Doctor and Patient*. Baltimore, MD: Johns Hopkins University Press.

Veatch R.M. (2009) *Patient, Heal Thyself: How the New Medicine Puts the Patient in Charge*. Oxford: Oxford University Press.

Wennberg J.E. (2010) *Tracking Medicine: A Researcher's Quest to Understand Health Care*. Oxford: Oxford University Press.

5 | Strengthening self-care

Overview

Here we consider the patients' role in self-care and the management of long-term conditions. After explaining these concepts and the important place of chronic conditions within the spectrum of disease, we look at the theoretical models that underpin various strategies for helping patients to manage their care effectively. Practical methods examined include self-management education courses and integrated clinical support, care planning, record access and personal health budgets.

Managing minor illness

Self-care is the most prevalent form of healthcare. Most of us cope with minor illnesses without recourse to professional help. We spend far more time looking after ourselves than being under the care of health professionals and the actions that we take to recognize, treat and manage our own health problems are a crucial determinant of the demand for professionally provided healthcare.

Consultation rates have risen in recent years. In 1995 the average patient in the UK had 3.9 primary care consultations per year, but by 2008 this had risen to 5.5 per year (Hippisley-Cox and Vinogradova 2009). Overall, consultations with primary care doctors and nurses in England increased by an estimated 44 per cent between 1998 and 2008. Health professionals often complain that they have to deal with too many consultations about trivial issues that do not require their help. The Department of Health has estimated that 40 per cent of GP time is spent dealing with minor, self-treatable illnesses that people could have managed themselves (Department of Health 2005b). However, based on the average consultation length of 11.7 minutes (Department of Health 2007) the average person spends not much more than an hour per year in the direct care of a health professional. The rest of the time they look after themselves. This simple fact is often overlooked in discussions about health policy, which tend to overemphasize the contribution of organized health services and underplay the individual's role in self-care.

Not all health problems reach the attention of doctors. Hannay used the metaphor of an iceberg to illustrate the point that health professionals, even those working in 'first contact' care such as general practice, see only a small fraction of the afflictions that could potentially trigger a consultation (Hannay 1980). In his Glasgow population study, even potentially serious symptoms were often managed at home or by seeking advice from a relative or friend, rather than going to see the doctor. These 'iceberg' cases outnumbered the trivial reasons for seeking professional help, when medical advice was not really necessary, by more than two to one.

People consult their doctors more readily nowadays than in the 1970s when Hannay carried out his study but the illness iceberg has not disappeared, although it is possible that professionals see a greater proportion of it than previously. It is still the case that some serious health problems are missed altogether or treated too late because people are reluctant to 'bother the doctor'. For example, men are often more reluctant to seek medical advice than women, and people from lower socio-economic groups are more likely to put off going to the GP than those from more advantaged sections of the population. Delays in consultation may be one explanation for the fact that the UK's cancer survival rates are worse than those in some other Western developed countries (Austoker et al. 2009).

The factors driving up consultation rates include social and demographic change, with more elderly people in the population, many of whom live alone; smaller and more dispersed family units leading to a loss of advice and support from relatives experienced in managing health problems; greater awareness of and concern about health issues due to extensive media coverage; and improved access to primary care making it easier to see a doctor or nurse quite quickly.

Support for self-care

Strengthening people's capacity to self-manage their health is a central part of government's attempts to control the demand for healthcare. Failure to support people's self-care efforts can encourage unnecessary dependency on professionals, leading to increased demand for expensive healthcare resources (Wanless 2002). It has been suggested that better self-care support could reduce GP consultations by up to 40 per cent, A&E visits and hospital admissions by up to 50 per cent, and outpatient visits by up to 17 per cent (Department of Health 2005b). The Self Care Campaign has estimated that the NHS spends around two billion pounds each year on treating minor conditions that do not need professional help (Self Care Campaign 2010).

With the aim of increasing people's capacity, confidence and efficacy for self-care and reducing unnecessary use of NHS resources, the Department of Health in England has encouraged investment in the following initiatives:

- provision of health information and advice
- health education
- self-care skills training

- first aid training in schools
- self-diagnostic tools, self-monitoring devices and self-care equipment
- multi-media self-care facilities and information materials
- individualized care plans
- patient access to medical records
- peer support networks
- public participation in design of local self-care programmes
- education of public and practitioners to change attitudes and behaviours towards self-care
- training practitioners to support self-care
- development of shared-care partnerships between professionals and public.

Whether these interventions will be sufficient to stem the rising demand for healthcare remains to be seen. In the meantime, initiatives such as these are needed to help ameliorate the effects of chronic disease and long-term conditions. In the rest of this chapter we examine the potential for improving self-management of these conditions.

The importance of chronic disease

Much self-care consists of the day-to-day management of long-term and chronic illnesses, such as asthma, diabetes and arthritis, also known as long-term conditions. Around 17 million people in the UK live with a long-term condition, some with more than one, including an estimated three out of every five people aged over 60. This proportion is set to rise by nearly a quarter over the next 25 years, the consequence of an ageing population. World-wide, 60 per cent of deaths are due to chronic diseases, with the main causes of mortality being cardiovascular disease (mainly heart disease and stroke), cancer (now classified as a chronic condition), chronic respiratory diseases (such as chronic obstructive pulmonary disease (COPD) and asthma), and diabetes (World Health Organization 2005).

In the UK, chronic diseases account for 85 per cent of all deaths, and people with these conditions use 52 per cent of all GP appointments, 65 per cent of all outpatient appointments and 72 per cent of all inpatient bed days (Department of Health 2004). The treatment and care of those with long-term conditions accounts for nearly 70 per cent of NHS expenditure on primary and secondary care. People with a long-term condition that affects their day-to-day activity are more than twice as likely to be out of work compared to those without long-term conditions. It has been estimated that the UK economy stands to lose roughly £16 billion over the next 10 years through premature deaths due to heart disease, stroke and diabetes.

The causes of chronic diseases have been summarized by the World Health Organization (WHO) as consisting of underlying socio-economic, cultural, political and environmental factors, modifiable health behaviours or risk factors and non-modifiable factors such as age or heredity, and intermediate risk factors such as raised blood pressure or obesity (World Health Organization 2005) (Figure 5.1).

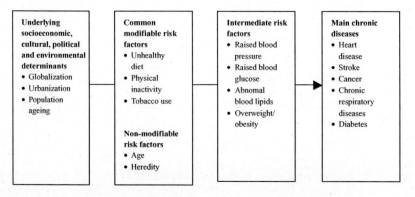

Source: Reproduced from the World Health Organization (2005) with permission

Figure 5.1 Main causes of chronic disease

Chronic diseases are now the leading cause of mortality in both rich and poor countries, so WHO has stressed the urgent need for governments, health organizations and individuals to take action to prevent and reduce the risk factors. Strategies to encourage people to adopt healthy lifestyles are essential to reduce the burden of chronic disease.

Self-management of long-term conditions

Self-management is what most people with long-term chronic conditions do all the time. They manage their daily lives and cope with the effects of their condition as best they can, for the most part without any intervention from professionals. Self-management has been defined as:

> The individual's ability to manage the symptoms, treatment, physical and social consequences and lifestyle changes inherent in living with a chronic condition.
>
> (Barlow et al. 2002: 178)

When people with chronic conditions seek professional advice, they need appropriate help and support to enhance their self-management skills. For example, people with asthma must know when to use their inhalers, people with diabetes must monitor their blood glucose levels, and people with arthritis need to learn how to cope with the pain and, where possible, how to ameliorate it. Most people with chronic conditions can benefit from modifying their lifestyles; for example, giving up smoking, losing weight, taking more exercise and eating a healthier diet. They also have to cope with the emotional impact of having a long-term condition and the practical effects on their daily lives.

Health professionals have a key role in supporting self-management (Mulligan et al. 2009). The types of support required may include the following:

- **Information**: about the disease, treatment or management options, and preventing exacerbations.
- **Education**: about effective self-management and behaviour change.
- **Self-monitoring**: being aware of symptoms and the factors that can modify them.
- **Skills training**: for example, how to carry out technical tasks such as testing blood glucose levels for diabetes, how to monitor peak flow for asthma, and how to adjust medication levels.
- **Behaviour change**: how to modify existing behaviours or adopt new ones and how to maintain changes.
- **Challenging unhelpful beliefs**: including beliefs about the causes of illness and what people can or cannot do to improve their condition.
- **Managing emotions**: how to cope with the impact of their illness and its effect on their emotions; for example, dealing with anxiety and depression.

Care planning

Surveys suggest that many patients do not get enough support from health professionals to self-manage effectively. For example, an international survey by the Commonwealth Fund asked people with complex health needs if they had been given a written plan to help them manage their care at home (Schoen et al. 2009) (Figure 5.2).

In all the countries apart from the USA, more than half of those who responded said they had not been given a plan. Of course, not everyone wants this type of help. A study in England of guided self-management plans for asthma found that participants were generally ambivalent about their usefulness and relevance, and few patients made consistent use of their own plan (Jones et al. 2000). Nevertheless, there is evidence that the vast majority of those with long-term conditions do want to play an active part in managing their condition and most welcome any support they can get. In a survey of people with long-term conditions, 82 per cent said they already play an active role in their care but would like to do more, more than 90 per cent were interested in being more active self-carers, and more than 75 per cent said that if they had guidance and support from a professional or peer they would feel far more confident about taking care of their own health (Department of Health 2005a).

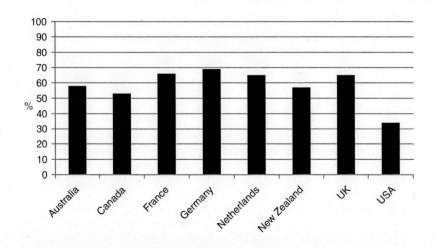

Source: 2008 Commonwealth Fund International Health Policy Survey of Sicker Adults. Reproduced with permission from the Commonwealth Fund

Figure 5.2 People with complex health needs who had not been given a written self-management plan

The Chronic Care Model

Policy-makers in many countries are now seeking ways to shift resources into the community and away from dependence on the expensive hospital sector in an effort to deal more effectively with long-term chronic problems and disabilities. The Chronic Care Model developed by Ed Wagner and his colleagues in the USA has been highly influential internationally (Wagner 1998) (Figure 5.3).

At the heart of the model is an informed and activated patient supported by a well-prepared, proactive primary care team. Recognizing that the health-care needs of chronically ill people may be different from those of people with acute conditions, the emphasis is on empowering them to manage their own health and healthcare. The role of the health professional is to provide effective self-management support by acknowledging the patient's central role in their own care and enhancing their confidence and skills. This can be achieved by a collaborative approach that involves working with them to define problems, establish goals, create treatment plans and providing help to implement any lifestyle changes deemed necessary; for example, smoking cessation, increased exercise and dietary change. The health system must be designed to support this approach, with an emphasis on proactive inter-ventions to keep people as healthy as possible, instead of just responding reactively when they are sick – a 'wellness' service rather than a 'sickness' service. Care should be evidence based and focused on interventions known

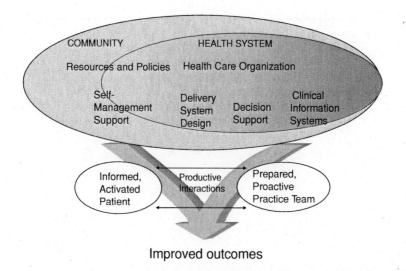

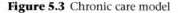

Improved outcomes

Source: Reproduced from Wagner (1998) with permission from the American College of Physicians

Figure 5.3 Chronic care model

to be effective. Information and decision support is required for both professionals and patients, including sharing practice guidelines so that patients understand the principles behind their care. Community resources such as local voluntary organizations and patient groups are a key component of the model, which is embedded in a population approach to health promotion.

Ideally self-management education and support should be integrated into the health system and used alongside other strategies for helping people with long-term conditions. The key is to target interventions appropriately, so that those who need intensive support from health professionals receive it, and those who could benefit from self-management support (the majority of people with long-term conditions) receive that. Various analytical tools are available to help target appropriate support to each level of need. For example, case-finding algorithms, such as the Patients at Risk of Re-hospitalisation (PARR) tool and the Combined Predictive Model, can be used to analyse data across a population to identify those in need of intensive, regular one-to-one support from a case manager to keep them out of hospital and those who may need less intensive intervention and self-management support (King's Fund, New York University and Health Dialog 2009).

Following the lead set by Kaiser Permanente in the USA, the Chronic Care Model is often represented by a pyramid indicating the levels of support required by different sub-groups (Figure 5.4).

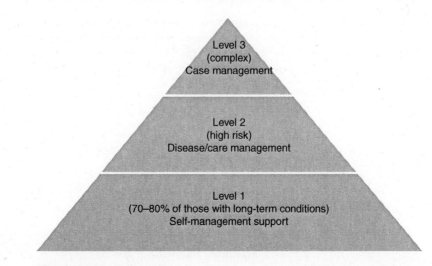

Figure 5.4 Pyramid of care

People at the top of the pyramid, often elderly, frail, and with multiple chronic problems and disabilities, are likely to require intensive support and multiple services coordinated by a case manager. Those at Level 2 may have more than one chronic condition requiring extensive medical input, but they can also benefit from self-management support. The vast majority of those with long-term conditions – Level 1 in the pyramid – will manage largely on their own, with appropriate self-management support when needed. Ideally this support should come from a well-managed, integrated health system where care is truly patient-centred and coordinated effectively to produce better health outcomes (Curry and Ham 2010).

Collaborative care

The Chronic Care Model suggests that collaborative relationships between clinicians and patients are key to encouraging better management of long-term conditions. Many strategies to promote collaborative care have been found to be effective (Bodenheimer 2003; Tsai et al. 2005). All include careful elicitation of the patient's view of his or her problems, concerns, values and preferences; sensitive sharing of relevant evidence-based information by health professionals; and discussion to find common ground. The model reflects an explicit shift in control to the patient, so it demands a culture change on the part of practitioners. Professionals are urged to stop believing that their goal is to increase patients' compliance to whatever they choose to recommend, and instead to increase the patient's capacity to make informed decisions:

We (and others) felt that a more appropriate and realistic purpose for diabetes patient education was to increase the learner's freedom/autonomy (i.e. one's capacity to make informed decisions) rather than increase the learner's conformity/compliance (i.e. one's willingness to follow the instructions of those in authority).

(Anderson and Funnell 2010: 278)

The five A's paradigm, derived from smoking cessation research and now commonly applied in chronic disease self-management programmes, codifies the professional's role as follows (Glasgow et al. 2006):

- **Assess** knowledge, behaviours and confidence routinely.
- **Advise** from scientific evidence and present information.
- **Agree** on goals and treatment plan for improving self-management.
- **Assist** in overcoming barriers.
- **Arrange** helpful services.

Chronic care system

The Chronic Care Model emphasizes the fact that self-management at the level of the individual patient requires a supportive culture at the organizational, community and health system levels. At the organizational level this requires effective multi-disciplinary teamwork, high-quality primary care, and effective integration of primary and secondary care (Curry and Ham 2010). At the community level it means strengthening prevention and tackling inequalities, as well as mobilizing other community resources, including housing, employment and social care services and the voluntary sector (Frosch et al. 2010). At the system level it means shifting the focus of attention and the investment of resources from treatment services in acute hospitals towards primary care and prevention (Samb et al. 2010).

Ham has outlined 10 characteristics of a high-performing chronic care system (Ham 2010):

1   **Universal coverage** – in other words, access to healthcare for all, funded either out of taxation or by some form of universal insurance. The importance of this point has been recognized in almost all developed countries except the USA.
2   **Healthcare that is free at the point of use** – so that no one is deterred from seeking appropriate care because of its cost.
3   **Focus on prevention** – not just on treating illness.
4   **Support self-management** – by acknowledging the role played by patients and their families and providing effective help to strengthen this.
5   **Prioritize primary care** – because most chronic disease management takes place in primary care.

6 **Emphasize population management** – by using analytical tools to stratify people with chronic diseases according to their risk and offering support commensurate with this risk.

7 **Integrate primary and secondary care** – to enable primary care teams to access specialist advice and support when needed.

8 **Use information technology** – to develop disease registers, to stratify the population according to risk, to promote better communication between professionals, to inform patients, to coordinate care, to improve safety and to support people at home.

9 **Coordinate care effectively** – especially for people with multiple conditions through health coaching and support by nurse specialists, and by integration with social care services.

10 **Develop a strategic approach to change** – by recognizing the cumulative effect of the above initiatives and moving forward on several fronts at once.

Theoretical underpinnings

The principles of self-management have been developed in a number of theoretical models, mostly from the fields of psychology and behavioural science. These focus on understanding the factors that shape behaviour and those that might help people make the necessary adaptations to improve their health and ability to cope with illness and disability. Of these, it is Bandura's Social Cognitive theory (Bandura 1977), Prochaska and DiClemente's 'Stages of Change' transtheoretical model (Prochaska and Diclemente 1992), and Leventhal's Self-Regulation theory (Leventhal et al. 1998) that are most widely referred to.

Bandura described the concept of self-efficacy, which refers to an individual's belief in their capacity to successfully learn and perform a specific behaviour. A strong sense of self-efficacy leads to a feeling of control, and willingness to take on and persist with new and difficult tasks. When applied to health, this theory suggests that people are empowered and motivated to manage their health problems when they feel confident about their ability to achieve this goal. So interventions for improving self-care should focus on confidence-building and equipping patients with the tools (knowledge and skills) to set personal goals and develop effective strategies for achieving them.

The Stages of Change model, which was developing to inform strategies to help people give up smoking, suggests that behaviour change involves transition through several stages – *pre-contemplation* (has no immediate intention to change), *contemplation* (intends to change behaviour within the next six months), *preparation* (has started to prepare for change within the next month), *action* (has begun to change) and *maintenance* (has managed to sustain change for more than six months). The model implies that attempts to encourage behaviour change should start by assessing which stage the individual has reached and tailor the intervention accordingly.

Self-Regulation theory focuses on people's mental representations of their illness or condition, how they make sense of this, and the adaptations or coping strategies they develop. It focuses on people's cognitive and emotional responses to health threats and the feedback loops they use as active problem-solvers in dealing with these. If health professionals understand an individual's personal response to their condition, they may be better placed to help them manage it.

Each of these theories has been invoked in the development of strategies for providing self-management support. We now look at some of these strategies and what is known about their effects.

Self-management education

People with chronic conditions; for example depression, eating disorders, asthma, arthritis and hypertension, have benefited from short (usually six weekly sessions) lay-led self-management education courses where they learn from other people with the same chronic condition (Lorig et al. 2001). Often run by voluntary organizations, participants in the courses learn how to:

- set goals and make action plans
- problem-solve
- develop their communication skills
- manage their emotions
- pace daily activities
- manage relationships with family, friends and work colleagues
- communicate with health and social care professionals
- find other healthcare resources in the community
- understand the importance of exercise, keeping active and healthy eating
- manage fatigue, sleep, pain, anger and depression.

In England the Expert Patient Programme runs self-management courses based on the chronic disease self-management programme originally developed by Kate Lorig and her colleagues from Stanford University, California. This model has been widely adopted internationally, with courses running in countries as diverse as Australia, Barbados, Chile, Denmark, Guatemala, Japan, Peru, Russia, Singapore, South Korea and Taiwan.

This type of self-help education can bring benefits in terms of improvements in knowledge, coping behaviour, adherence to treatment recommendations and self-efficacy, and modest short-term improvements in pain, disability, fatigue and depression (Chodosh et al. 2005; Foster et al. 2007). However, few studies of chronic disease self-management education programmes have looked at long-term outcomes and there is dispute about its cost-effectiveness. Despite claims that this type of approach can reduce demand for medical care, studies have produced conflicting results and the effects are likely to be small. One trial that included an assessment of the cost-effectiveness of six-session lay-led self-management courses for people with arthritis found no impact on numbers of GP consultations and no evidence of improved cost-effectiveness, but patients' anxiety levels and perceived self-efficacy improved following the courses (Buszewicz et al. 2006; Patel et al. 2009). Another study also found significant improvements in self-efficacy and energy among Expert Patient Programme participants (Kennedy et al. 2007). There was no measurable impact on their subsequent use of health services, but the authors concluded that the benefits of the intervention meant it was likely to be cost-effective at a societal level.

The key to success lies in encouraging participation by those who can benefit most, in particular younger people, those who lack confidence to manage their condition, and those who are finding it particularly hard to cope (Reeves et al. 2008). Particular effort may be required to recruit these types of people into self-management education programmes since other pressures in their lives may inhibit their ability to attend courses. Indeed courses may not be the best way to provide self-management support to such groups – other strategies may be more appropriate.

Integrated self-management support

Self-management education seems to work best when it is integrated into primary and secondary healthcare systems and the learning is reinforced by professionals. Many professionally led self-management education programmes are aimed at specific patient groups. For example, people with diabetes have been seen to gain health benefits from self-management education, leading to improved clinical indicators and better quality of life outcomes (Cochran and Conn 2008; Deakin et al. 2005; Ismail et al. 2004; Norris et al. 2002). There is evidence that these programmes can be cost-effective, so therapeutic education programmes specially designed for people with type 2 diabetes have been recommended for widespread use (Albano et al. 2008; Gillett et al. 2010).

The Year of Care in diabetes is a pilot programme that was launched in response to a national patient survey that showed that many diabetes patients in England were not being actively encouraged to participate in planning or managing their care (Diabetes UK 2010). The programme aims to go further than simply providing education to actively involve people with diabetes in deciding, agreeing and owning how their diabetes is managed. The idea is to transform the annual review, which often just checks that particular tests have been carried out, into a genuinely collaborative consultation by encouraging patients to share information with their healthcare team about their concerns, their experience of living with diabetes, and any services or support they might need. Both the patient and the healthcare team will then jointly agree the priorities or goals and the actions to take in response to these.

This type of approach, which aims to rebalance the relationship between patients and professionals, is backed up by a body of evidence suggesting it could achieve better outcomes at lower cost. Discussion and collaboration is key – initiatives that rely on providing information alone are not effective, although they can be helpful for building background knowledge. Professionals must help patients to engage with the information, recognizing their experience of dealing with their health condition and being ready to review alternative strategies with them (Protheroe et al. 2008). Written information to reinforce educational messages given in clinical consultations, for example, self-management guidelines, can also be helpful.

This type of interactive approach can also be delivered by computer. For example, the Expert Patient Programme has been developed as a web module with email reminders and it appears to work well (Lorig et al. 2008). Web-based packages that combine health information with social support, decision support or behaviour change support have been developed for people with chronic conditions such as asthma, diabetes, eating disorders and urinary incontinence. Evidence from systematic reviews of computer-based interactive applications found that patients' knowledge and abilities increased, they felt they had better social support, and their health behaviours and clinical outcomes improved (Kaltenthaler et al. 2002; Murray et al. 2005).

The most effective self-management education programmes are those that are longer and more intensive, are well-integrated into the health system, and where the learning is reinforced by health professionals during regular follow-up. Efforts need to be focused on providing opportunities for patients to develop practical skills and the confidence to self-manage their health. Hands-on participative learning styles are better than traditional didactic teaching.

Supporting people in their own homes

Telephone health coaching – providing people with advice and support over the phone as a component of disease management systems – is becoming popular in the USA and elsewhere as a means of providing self-management support. Usually provided by nurses working from call centres, it uses motivational interviewing techniques (see Chapter 3) to support individual lifestyle change, treatment adherence, shared decision-making and self-management (Rollnick et al. 2002). Evidence about the effects of telephone coaching on outcomes for patients with chronic disease is currently limited, but studies showing beneficial effects are beginning to emerge. For example, it has been shown to reduce coronary heart disease risk factors and improve medication adherence (Jelinek et al. 2009) and it reduces deaths and hospitalizations for people with chronic heart failure (Inglis et al. 2010). A large randomized controlled trial in the USA compared population-based telephone health coaching at two levels of intensity, basic and enhanced (Wennberg et al. 2010). The health coaches provided advice on behaviour change, motivational interviewing, decision aids and decision support. This led to a reduction in admission rates of 10 per cent among those who received enhanced support and their healthcare costs were 3.6 per cent lower than those of the usual support group.

Many patient organizations provide telephone advice lines and these receive large numbers of calls. There is little robust evidence on their effects, but peer-to-peer telephone support undoubtedly helps some patients and their carers obtain information and practical assistance, as well as being a forum to share experiences and feelings with people in a similar situation (Dale et al. 2008). Proactive telephone messaging also has great potential as an inexpensive way to encourage behaviour change (Cole-Lewis and Kershaw 2010). For example, simple text messages sent to patients in Kenya via their mobile phones proved to be effective in improving adherence to HIV treatment (Lester et al. 2010).

Telecare is a term used to describe a range of information and communication technologies to support the delivery of care directly to people in their own homes. Other terms, often used interchangeably, include telehealth and telemonitoring. These technologies are often used as a means of helping frail elderly people or those with physical or learning disabilities to remain living independently in their own homes as long as possible, while others provide advice and motivational support to a range of people with long-term conditions. They are distinguished from telemedicine which refers to applications designed for use by health professionals to facilitate remote use of specialist advice and services.

Telecare includes a range of technologies, from devices that enable transmission of information through phone lines to sophisticated machines to monitor people's 'vital signs' and computers that control features in a person's home. They can be used to provide information and support, to monitor safety and security, and to measure physiological parameters while people go about their daily lives (Audit Commission 2004). Examples include telephone or web-based information systems providing reminders and other self-management education and advice; pendant alarms or movement detectors to alert community support services if an elderly person has had a fall and cannot get up; and ambulatory blood pressure monitors or electronic skin-contact sensors that can download vital signs (physiological indicators) for the person to review themselves and alert a health professional when necessary, or to provide remote access for direct monitoring by health professionals.

Again, robust evidence on the effectiveness of these technologies is relatively sparse, but vital signs monitoring and telephone follow-up by nurses appears to be beneficial (Barlow et al. 2007). There is evidence from the Veterans Health Administration in the USA of significant reductions in hospital admissions as a result of providing telecare support, coupled with high rates of patient satisfaction (Darkins et al. 2008). Telemonitoring has also been shown to have beneficial effects for people with heart failure (Inglis et al. 2010). In 2010 it was estimated that around 1.7 million people in England were using some form of telecare, but this was mostly pendant alarms, with only about 5,000 people receiving home-based remote monitoring for conditions such as heart failure, chronic obstructive pulmonary disorder and diabetes (Clark and Goodwin 2010).

New technologies enable patients to carry out tasks that could previously be done only by professionals. For example, with self-monitoring systems people can monitor their own blood pressure, measure their blood glucose or administer anticoagulation therapy and adjust their medication as necessary(Garcia-Alamino et al. 2010; Welschen et al. 2005). People who use these technologies can achieve results that are equal to or better than those achieved by health professionals, but not all patients want or are able to do it.

There is also interest in using electronic social networking sites such as Facebook to provide peer support for people with long-term conditions. There is little evidence as yet that this type of 'virtual community' has an impact on health outcomes, but it may help to improve people's sense of social support (Eysenbach et al. 2004).

Record access

Giving patients access to their medical records – either by making it possible for them to read and review these, or by encouraging them to hold their own copy – has been shown to increase knowledge and understanding and many patients find it empowering. For example, studies of women undergoing maternity care found that patients valued the opportunity to hold their own case notes – it gave them a greater sense of control and the records were less likely to get lost (Brown and Smith 2007). Patient-held records have also been used in cancer care, where they have been welcomed by patients but have failed to generate much interest among health professionals (Gysels et al. 2007). While patients who hold copies of their records usually appreciate the opportunity, health professionals sometimes resent the idea because of concerns about increased paperwork, duplication of records, and the possibility that patients may misinterpret the information causing them to become upset or anxious.

Even if patients are not given a copy of their record to keep, many appreciate having the opportunity to look at it. Patients in the UK have had the right to read their medical records since 1998, though few have exercised it. Record access can help patients manage their care, especially when coupled with targeted information and decision support (Royal College of General Practitioners 2010). Despite this, patients have often found that health professionals can be obstructive when they ask to see their medical records. In 2003 the Department of Health in England issued guidelines recommending that letters written by one health professional to another should be copied to the patient, or the parent or legal guardian where appropriate (Department of Health 2003). They listed the following benefits of copying letters between professionals and patients:

- **More trust between patients and professionals**: increased openness and trust between professionals and patients.
- **Better informed patients**: patients and carers have a better understanding of their condition and how they can help themselves.
- **Better decisions**: patients are more informed and better able to make decisions about treatment options.
- **Better compliance**: patients who understand the reasons for taking medication or treatment are more likely to follow advice.
- **More accurate records**: errors can be spotted and corrected by the patient.
- **Better consultations**: patients are better prepared and less anxious, leading to better discussions and improved comprehension.
- **Health promotion**: the letters can be used to reinforce advice on self-care and behaviour change.
- **Clearer letters between professionals**: improves clarity of communication for both professionals and patients.

Notwithstanding this official endorsement, more than half of patients in England discharged from hospital in 2009 said they did not receive copies of letters written about them (Care Quality Commission 2010). The majority of those who did receive the letters said they were written in a way they could understand. Some hospital consultants now address their letters to the patient, with a copy to the GP, a practice that helpfully serves to underline the patient's key role in managing their own care.

In theory electronic records should be easier to share with patients than paper ones. This practice is widespread in Denmark, where patients can electronically access all of their medical information including medical records, test results and hospital discharge letters. They can also schedule appointments, renew prescriptions, and access advice out-of-hours when they need it. Systems are being introduced in the UK to offer similar facilities. Implementation of hospital-based systems has been slow, but some GPs have been offering electronic record access for several years. A study in one practice to explore patients' experience of using an electronic record system found that most patients responded very positively, but 70 per cent found at least one error or omission in their record (Pyper et al. 2004). Most of these were trivial, but some errors or omissions could have had an adverse impact on their clinical care. The patients were able to ensure that the errors were recognized and corrected.

Now that Internet access and email messaging is so common, many patients want the opportunity to seek medical advice using these means (Ye et al. 2010). In some integrated health systems in the USA, patients make extensive use of email messaging to communicate with their doctors. For example, in Kaiser Permanente this has led to reductions in outpatient visits and telephone contacts, as well as improved convenience for patients (Liang 2007). Following consultations, Kaiser patients can print a summary sheet that lists their medications, educational information and doctors' notes. Proponents argue that accessing their records via a website helps patients, especially those with long-term conditions, to adhere to treatment recommendations and better communicate their needs. In some settings they can also access online health information and risk assessment tools that are designed to help improve understanding and, where necessary, stimulate behaviour change. But electronic communication between doctors and patients has been slow to take off in most European countries, including the UK (Santana et al. 2010).

Personal health budgets

Since 1996 people in the UK who have been assessed as being eligible for social care support have had the option to take a direct cash payment to purchase the support they choose, instead of relying on social care professionals to organize it for them. The aim of the scheme is to empower people to have more choice and control over their care. Similar schemes are in operation in many other countries, including Australia, Belgium, Canada, France, Germany, Italy, the Netherlands, Sweden and the USA (Carr and Robbins 2009). Evaluations have found that social care users are very positive about the schemes when they are given sufficient support to use them effectively (Alakeson 2010).

Buoyed by this success, the government in England decided to extend the scheme to healthcare, with the launch of 70 pilot sites around the country. Focused in particular on those with long-term conditions, including mental healthcare and end-of-life care, the hope is that this will improve responsiveness to patients, while at the same time leading to better targeting of resources and better health outcomes. However, the policy carries a number of risks, including the possibility that some people might find the extra responsibility hard to handle, that they might misspend the money on services or equipment that confer no benefit, or that it will increase inequalities because it disproportionately benefits people from the most advantaged groups (Jones et al. 2010). Despite general enthusiasm for the concept in principle, there is considerable scepticism about the ability of the NHS to cope with such a fundamental change in organizing and paying for services, especially during a time of financial stringency (National Mental Health Development Unit and Mental Health Network 2009).

There are at least three ways in which personal health budgets can operate (Department of Health 2009):

1 People can be given notional budgets where no money actually changes hands, but they liaise with their doctor or care manager to influence the way the funds are spent within a fixed budget limit.

2   They are given a real budget that is managed on their behalf by a third party, possibly a voluntary organization or patient association.
3   They receive actual cash in the form of a direct payment to buy the services they and their doctor or care manager decide they need. They have to show what they spend it on, but they are responsible for buying and managing the services themselves.

The reports on personal care budgets (or self-directed care as it is known in the USA) include many heart-warming case studies showing how people's lives have been transformed by the empowering experience of holding their own budget, many of whom have both health and social care needs; for example, the cancer patient who used her personal budget to make several adaptations to her home to avoid the need for institutional care, and the mental health patient who employed her own care staff because she had particular language and religious needs (Tyson et al. 2010).

Since individuals do not tend to think of their needs as being easily compartmentalized into social or healthcare, it makes sense to think of expanding the scheme to cover other aspects of their lives. However, initial experience has identified a number of challenges faced by the health budget pilot sites. These include how to determine costs and set budgets; how to find the additional funding necessary to set up the scheme; how to determine the scope of the scheme; that is, which services can be purchased and which should be ruled out; how to manage risk; how to organize care planning, providing sufficient support to the individual budget holder to allow for true personalization of services; how to ensure the scheme is equitable and does not create an imbalance in local services; how to ensure sufficient choice of services; how to ensure the scheme is well managed and accountable; how to achieve the required culture shift among health professionals; how to integrate health and social care budgets and services; and how to manage the impact on the workforce involved in delivering the services (Jones et al. 2010).

The personal budgets pilot schemes are being independently evaluated so there will be an opportunity to learn whether these challenges can be overcome satisfactorily. The goal of making services more flexible and personalized is highly attractive, but whether giving people individual budgets is the best way to achieve this is as yet unproven.

Evidence on what works

A very large number of studies have been carried out to evaluate different types of self-management support in specific groups of patients; for example, those with arthritis, asthma, cancer, heart disease, COPD, diabetes, epilepsy, HIV/AIDS, hypertension, mental illness and stroke. Many of these have been summarized in systematic reviews. An overview of 124 systematic reviews of self-management interventions drew the following general conclusions about what is known and not known in relation to the effects of supporting self-management in people with long-term conditions (Picker Institute Europe 2010).

1 **Impact on knowledge**: most of the reviews that looked at the effects of informing and educating patients found that it was possible to improve people's understanding of their condition and their recall of key facts, but information alone was not sufficient to impact on symptoms or behaviours.

2 **Impact on coping skills**: the reviews looked at a wide range of conditions and outcome measures so it is quite hard to summarize these, but there is a substantial body of evidence showing that it is possible to improve people's coping skills and their confidence to manage their condition. However, most studies have looked at short-term outcomes rather than long-term effects, so there are still questions about what needs to be done to ensure results are sustained over the longer term.

3 **Impact on health behaviour and health status**: the studies show mixed results depending on the type of intervention and patient group. For example, short-term improvements in health status have been observed following arthritis self-management education, but these were not sustained in the longer term. Studies of asthma self-management education found mixed results, as did those for cancer patients. Health education and stress management programmes can improve health behaviours (e.g. smoking cessation) and outcomes for patients with coronary heart disease. There is as yet little evidence of improvements resulting from self-management support for patients with COPD. Most reviews, but not all, found improvements in blood glucose control as a result of self-management support for people with diabetes. Self-management support can improve adherence to treatment recommendations and reduce seizure frequency among people with epilepsy. People with HIV/AIDS can benefit from self-management support leading to improved treatment adherence and less unsafe sex. Home blood pressure monitoring plus counselling, education and reminders can lead to better blood pressure control among people with hypertension. Collaborative care techniques can improve treatment adherence and reduce depression, but there is only limited evidence that educational programmes had a beneficial effect on people with psychological problems.

4 **Impact on service utilization and costs**: few studies have looked at cost-effectiveness. There is some evidence of reduction in hospitalization rates, unscheduled visits to the doctor and days off work or school as a result of self-management education and care planning for people with asthma. There is evidence that self-monitoring of oral anticoagulation is as effective as specialist management and superior to GP care, but wide adoption could be quite costly. Most, though not all, economic analyses find that diabetes self-management training is cost-effective. There is conflicting evidence of an effect on service use following generic lay-led self-management programmes; any effect is likely to be marginal and

disease-specific programmes may be more effective. Interactive computer-based technologies can improve outcomes and are likely to be cost-effective.

So there is evidence that self-management can be effective, but more research is needed on the best ways to support people with long-term conditions and how to translate the learning from these studies into the mainstream of clinical practice. The case for change is strong – chronic diseases constitute the major burden of ill-health – but tackling them effectively will require a significant culture change in the way healthcare is delivered, with more emphasis on prevention and a better coordinated, more integrated health system.

Summary

Patients play a key role in their own healthcare, so this fact deserves greater recognition and support than it has received hitherto. Supporting self-care should be an important component of any strategy to manage the demand for healthcare. Treating and managing chronic conditions accounts for a very considerable proportion of healthcare resources and expenditure is rising as a result of demographic change. Managing these conditions and living with them requires personalized care and effective strategies to promote better self-management. Given the right tools and support, the evidence shows that people with long-term conditions can be empowered to set their own self-management goals and implement appropriate strategies for meeting them. The role of health professionals in guiding patients through the process is crucial. The goal is patient autonomy, but responsibility for achieving this must be shared by patients and health professionals alike.

References

Alakeson, V. (2010) *International Developments in Self-directed Care*. New York: Commonwealth Fund.

Albano, M.G., Crozet, C. and d'Ivernois, J.F. (2008) Analysis of the 2004–2007 literature on therapeutic patient education in diabetes: results and trends, *Acta Diabetologica*, 45(4): 211–19.

Anderson, R.M. and Funnell, M.M. (2010) Patient empowerment: myths and misconceptions, *Patient Education and Counseling*, 79(3): 277–82.

Audit Commission (2004) *Implementing Telecare*. London: Audit Commission.

Austoker, J., Bankhead, C., Forbes, L.J., Atkins, L., Martin, F., Robb, K., Wardle, J. and Ramirez, A.J. (2009) Interventions to promote cancer awareness and early presentation: systematic review, *British Journal of Cancer*, 101(Suppl. 2): S31–S39.

Bandura, A. (1977) Self-efficacy: toward a unifying theory of behavioral change, *Psychological Review*, 84: 191.

Barlow, J., Singh, D., Bayer, S. and Curry, R. (2007) A systematic review of the benefits of home telecare for frail elderly people and those with long-term conditions, *Journal of Telemedicine and Telecare*, 13(4): 172–79.

Barlow, J., Wright, C., Sheasby, J., Turner, A. and Hainsworth, J. (2002) Self-management approaches for people with chronic conditions: a review, *Patient Education and Counseling*, 48(2): 177–87.

Bodenheimer, T. (2003) Interventions to improve chronic illness care: evaluating their effectiveness, *Disease Management*, 6(2): 63–71.

Brown, H.C. and Smith, H.J. (2007) Giving women their own case notes to carry during pregnancy, *Cochrane Database of Systematic Review*, vol. CD002856 no, 2.

Buszewicz, M., Rait, G., Griffin, M., Nazareth, I., Patel, A., Atkinson, A., Barlow, J. and Haines, A. (2006) Self management of arthritis in primary care: randomised controlled trial, *British Medical Journal*, 333(7574): 879.

Care Quality Commission (2010) *Inpatient Survey 2009*. Newcastle: Care Quality Commission.

Carr, S. and Robbins, D. (2009) *The Implementation of Individual Budget Schemes in Adult Social Care*. London: Social Care Institute for Excellence, Research Briefing no. 20.

Chodosh, J., Morton, S.C., Mojica, W., Maglione, M., Suttorp, M.J., Hilton, L., Rhodes, S. and Shekelle, P. (2005) Meta-analysis: chronic disease self-management programs for older adults, *Annals of Internal Medicine*, 143(6): 427–38.

Clark, M. and Goodwin, N. (2010) *Sustaining Innovation in Telehealth and Telecare*. London: King's Fund.

Cochran, J. and Conn, V.S. (2008) Meta-analysis of quality of life outcomes following diabetes self-management training, *The Diabetes Educator*, 34(5): 815–23.

Cole-Lewis, H. and Kershaw, T. (2010) Text messaging as a tool for behavior change in disease prevention and management, *Epidemiology Review*, 32(1): 56–69.

Curry, N. and Ham, C. (2010) *Clinical and Service Integration: The Route to Improved Outcomes*. London: King's Fund.

Dale, J., Caramlau, I.O., Lindenmeyer, A. and Williams, S.M. (2008) Peer Support Telephone Calls for Improving Health. *Cochrane Database of Systematic Review*, vol. no.: CD006903. DOI: 10.1002/14651858.CD006903.pub2.

Darkins, A., Ryan, P., Kobb, R., Foster, L., Edmonson, E., Wakefield, B. and Lancaster, A.E. (2008) Care coordination/home telehealth: the systematic implementation of health informatics, home telehealth, and disease management to support the care of veteran patients with chronic conditions, *Telemedicine Journal and e-health*, 14(10): 1118–26.

Deakin, T., McShane, C.E., Cade, J.E. and Williams, R.D. (2005) Group based training for self-management strategies in people with type 2 diabetes mellitus, *Cochrane Database of Systematic Review*, vol. 2, no.: CD003417.

Department of Health (2003) *Copying Letters to Patients: Good Practice Guidelines for Sharing Letters with Patients*. London: Department of Health.

Department of Health (2004) *Improving Chronic Disease Management*. London: Department of Health.

Department of Health (2005a) *Public Attitudes to Self Care: Baseline Survey*. London: Department of Health.

Department of Health (2005b) *Self Care – A Real Choice*. London: Department of Health.

Department of Health (2007) *2006/7 UK General Practice Workload Survey*. London: BMA, NHS Employers, Department of Health. The Information Centre.

Department of Health (2009) *Personal Health Budgets: First Steps*. London: Department of Health.

Diabetes UK (2010) *Year of Care for Diabetes*. Available online at www.diabetes.org.uk; accessed August 2010.

Eysenbach, G., Powell, J., Englesakis, M., Rizo, C. and Stern, A. (2004) Health related virtual communities and electronic support groups: systematic review of the effects of online peer to peer interactions, *British Medical Journal*, 328(7449): 1166.

Foster, G., Taylor, S.J., Eldridge, S.E., Ramsay, J. and Griffiths, C.J. (2007) Self-management education programmes by lay leaders for people with chronic conditions, *Cochrane Database of Systematic Review*, no. 4: CD005108.

Frosch, D.L., Rincon, D., Ochoa, S. and Mangione, C.M. (2010) Activating seniors to improve chronic disease care: results from a pilot intervention study, *Journal of the American Geriatrics Society*, 58(8): 1496–503.

Garcia-Alamino, J.M., Ward, A.M., Alonso-Coello, P., Perera, R., Bankhead, C., Fitzmaurice, D. and Heneghan, C.J. (2010) Self-monitoring and self-management of oral anticoagulation, *Cochrane Database of Systematic Review*, no. 4: CD003839.

Gillett, M., Dallosso, H.M., Dixon, S., Brennan, A., Carey, M.E., Campbell, M.J., Heller, S., Khunti, K., Skinner, T.C. and Davies, M.J. (2010) Delivering the diabetes education and self management for ongoing and newly diagnosed (DESMOND) programme for people with newly diagnosed type 2 diabetes: cost effectiveness analysis, *British Medical Journal*, 341: c4093.

Glasgow, R.E., Emont, S. and Miller, D.C. (2006) Assessing delivery of the five 'As' for patient-centred counseling, *Health Promotion International*, 21(3): 245–55.

Gysels, M., Richardson, A. and Higginson, I.J. (2007) Does the patient-held record improve continuity and related outcomes in cancer care: a systematic review, *Health Expectations*, 10(1): 75–91.

Ham, C. (2010) The ten characteristics of the high-performing chronic care system, *Health Economics, Policy and Law*, 5: 71–90.

Hannay, D.R. (1980) The 'iceberg' of illness and 'trivial' consultations, *Journal of the Royal College of General Practitioners*, 30: 551–54.

Hippisley-Cox, J. and Vinogradova, Y. (2009) *Trends in Consultation Rates in General Practice 1995–2008: Analysis of the QResearch Database*. London: Health and Social Care Information Centre,

Inglis, S.C., Clark, R.A., McAlister, F.A., Ball, J., Lewinter, C., Cullington, D., Stewart, S. and Cleland, J.G. (2010) Structured telephone support or telemonitoring programmes for patients with chronic heart failure, *Cochrane Database of Systematic Review*, no. 8: CD007228.

Ismail, K., Winkley, K. and Rabe-Hesketh, S. (2004) Systematic review and meta-analysis of randomised controlled trials of psychological interventions to improve glycaemic control in patients with type 2 diabetes, *The Lancet*, 363(9421): 1589–97.

Jelinek, M., Vale, M.J., Liew, D., Grigg, L., Dart, A., Hare, D.L. and Best, J.D. (2009) The COACH program produces sustained improvements in cardiovascular risk factors and adherence to recommended medications-two years follow-up, *Heart, Lung and Circulation*, 18(6): 388–92.

Jones, A., Pill, R. and Adams, S. (2000) Qualitative study of views of health professionals and patients on guided self management plans for asthma, *British Medical Journal*, 321(7275): 1507–10.

Jones, K., Caiels, J., Forder, J., Windle, K., Welch, E., Dolan, P., Glendinning, C. and King, D. (2010) *Early Experiences of Implementing Personal Health Budgets*. London: Department of Health.

Kaltenthaler, E., Shackley, P., Stevens, K., Beverley, C., Parry, G. and Chilcott, J. (2002) A systematic review and economic evaluation of computerised cognitive behaviour therapy for depression and anxiety, *Health Technology Assessment*, 6(22): 1–89.

Kennedy, A., Reeves, D., Bower, P., Lee, V., Middleton, E., Richardson, G., Gardner, C., Gately, C. and Rogers, A. (2007) The effectiveness and cost effectiveness of a national lay-led self care support programme for patients with long-term conditions: a pragmatic randomised controlled trial, *Journal of Epidemiology Community Health*, 61(3): 254–61.

King's Fund, New York University, and Health Dialog (2009) *Predicting and Reducing Re-admission to Hospital*. London: King's Fund.

Lester, R.T., Ritvo, P., Mills, E.J., Kariri, A., Karanja, S., Chung, M.H., Jack, W., Habyarimana, J., Sadatsafavi, M., Najafzadeh, M., Marra, C.A., Estambale, B., Ngugi, E., Ball, T.B., Thabane, L., Gelmon, L.J., Kimani, J., Ackers, M. and Plummer, F.A. (2010) Effects of a mobile phone short message service on antiretroviral treatment adherence in Kenya (WelTel Kenya1): a randomised trial, *The Lancet*, 376(9755): 1838–45.

Leventhal, H., Leventhal, E.A. and Contrada, R.J. (1998) Self-regulation, health and behavior: a perceptual-cognitive approach, *Psychology and Health*, 13: 717–33.

Liang, L.L. (2007) The use of IT/electronic medical records to improve care coordination, efficiency, and patient safety. Paper presented at the Commonwealth Fund and Nuffield Trust, 8th International Meeting on Quality of Health Care.

Lorig, K.R., Ritter, P., Stewart, A.L., Sobel, D.S., Brown, B.W., Jr., Bandura, A., Gonzalez, V.M., Laurent, D.D. and Holman, H.R. (2001) Chronic disease self-management program: 2-year health status and health care utilization outcomes, *Medical Care*, 39(11): 1217–23.

Lorig, K.R., Ritter, P.L., Dost, A., Plant, K., Laurent, D.D. and McNeil, I. (2008) The Expert Patients Programme online, a 1-year study of an Internet-based self-management programme for people with long-term conditions, *Chronic Illness*, 4(4): 247–56.

Mulligan, K., Steed, L. and Newman, S. (2009) Different types and components of self-management interventions, in S. Newman, L. Steed and K. Mulligan (eds), *Chronic Physical Illness: Self-management and Behavioural Interventions*, 1st edn (pp. 64–77). Maidenhead: Open University Press.

Murray, E., Burns, J., See, T.S., Lai, R. and Nazareth, I. (2005) Interactive health communication applications for people with chronic disease, *Cochrane Database of Systematic Review*, no. 4: CD004274.

National Mental Health Development Unit and Mental Health Network (2009) *Shaping Personal Health Budgets: A View from the Top*. London: NHS Confederation.

Norris, S.L., Lau, J., Smith, S.J., Schmid, C.H. and Engelgau, M.M. (2002) Self-management education for adults with type 2 diabetes: a meta-analysis of the effect on glycemic control, *Diabetes Care*, 25(7): 1159–71.

Patel, A., Buszewicz, M., Beecham, J., Griffin, M., Rait, G., Nazareth, I., Atkinson, A., Barlow, J. and Haines, A. (2009) Economic evaluation of arthritis self management in primary care, *British Medical Journal*, 339: b3532.

Picker Institute Europe (2010) *Invest in Engagement: Self-management*. Available online at www.investinengagement.info, accessed 14 August 2010.

Prochaska, J.O. and Diclemente, C.C. (1992) Stages of change in the modification of problem behaviors, *Program Behaviour Modification*, 28: 183–218.

Protheroe, J., Rogers, A., Kennedy, A.P., Macdonald, W. and Lee, V. (2008) Promoting patient engagement with self-management support information: a qualitative meta-synthesis of processes influencing uptake, *Implementation Science*, 3: 44.

Pyper, C., Amery, J., Watson, M. and Crook, C. (2004) Patients' experiences when accessing their on-line electronic patient records in primary care, *British Journal of General Practice*, 54(498): 38–43.

Reeves, D., Kennedy, A., Fullwood, C., Bower, P., Gardner, C., Gately, C., Lee, V., Richardson, G. and Rogers, A. (2008) Predicting who will benefit from an Expert Patients Programme self-management course, *British Journal of General Practice*, 58(548): 198–203.

Rollnick, S., Miller, W.R. and Butler, C.C. (2002) *Motivational Interviewing: Preparing People to Change*, 2nd edn. New York: Guilford Press.

Royal College of General Practitioners (2010) *Enabling Patients to Access Electronic Health Records: Guidance for Health Professionals*. London: Royal College of General Practitioners.

Samb, B., Desai, N., Nishtar, S., Mendis, S., Bekedam, H., Wright, A., Hsu, J., Martiniuk, A., Celletti, F., Patel, K., Adshead, F., McKee, M., Evans, T., Alwan, A. and Etienne, C. (2010) Prevention and management of chronic disease: a litmus test for health-systems strengthening in low-income and middle-income countries, *The Lancet*, 376(9754): 1785–97.

Santana, S., Lausen, B., Bujnowska-Fedak, M., Chronaki, C., Kummervold, P.E., Rasmussen, J. and Sorensen, T. (2010) Online communication between doctors and patients in Europe: status and perspectives, *Journal of Medical Internet Research*, 12(2): e20.

Schoen, C., Osborn, R., How, S.K., Doty, M.M. and Peugh, J. (2009) In chronic condition: experiences of patients with complex health care needs, in eight countries, 2008, *Health Aff (Millwood)*, 28(1): w1–16.

Self Care Campaign (2010) *Self Care: An Ethical Imperative*. Available online at www.selfcarecampaign.org; accessed 8 August 2010.

Tsai, A.C., Morton, S.C., Mangione, C.M. and Keeler, E.B. (2005) A meta-analysis of interventions to improve care for chronic illnesses, *American Journal of Managed Care*, 11(8): 478–88.

Tyson, A., Brewis, R., Crosby, N., Hatton, C., Stansfield, J., Tomlinson, C., Waters, J. and Wood, A. (2010) *A Report on In Control's Third Phase: Evaluation and Learning 2008–9*. London: In Control Publications.

Wagner, E.H. (1998) Chronic disease management: what will it take to improve care for chronic illness?, *Effective Clinical Practice*, 1(1): 2–4.

Wanless, D. (2002) *Securing our Future Health: Taking a Long-term View*. London: HM Treasury.

Welschen, L.M., Bloemendal, E., Nijpels, G., Dekker, J.M., Heine, R.J., Stalman, W.A. and Bouter, L.M. (2005) Self-monitoring of blood glucose in patients with type 2 diabetes who are not using insulin, *Cochrane Database of Systematic Review*, no. 2: CD005060.

Wennberg, D.E., Marr, A., Lang, L., O'Malley, S. and Bennett, G. (2010) A randomized trial of a telephone care-management strategy, *The New England Journal of Medicine*, 363(13): 1245–55.

World Health Organization (2005) *Preventing Chronic Diseases: A Vital Investment*. Geneva: WHO.

Ye, J., Rust, G., Fry-Johnson, Y. and Strothers, H. (2010) E-mail in patient-provider communication: a systematic review, *Patient Education and Counseling*, 80(2): 266–73.

Further reading

Busse, R., Blümel, M., Scheller-Kreinsen, D., Zentner, A. (2010) *Tackling Chronic Disease in Europe: Strategies, Interventions and Challenges*. Copenhagen: Observatory Studies Series no. 20, World Health Organization.

Expert Patients Programme (2007) *Self-management of Long-term Health Conditions: A Handbook for People with Chronic Disease*. Boulder, CO: Bull Publishing Company.

Kleinman, A. (1988) *The Illness Narratives: Suffering, Healing and the Human Condition*. New York: Basic Books.

Newman, S., Steed, L. and Mulligan, K. (2009) *Chronic Physical Illness: Self-management and Behavioural Interventions*. Maidenhead: Open University Press.

6 Ensuring safer care

Overview

This chapter focuses on the patient's role in patient safety. After reviewing the general case for seeing patients as key players in promoting safer care, and discussing what should be done when things go wrong, we look at specific ways in which the patient's role could be significant: choosing safe providers, helping to reach an accurate diagnosis, participating in treatment decisions, contributing to safe medication use, participating in infection control initiatives, checking the accuracy of medical records, observing and checking care processes, reporting adverse events, practising effective self-care, and advocacy and feedback.

Patient safety

It has always been clear that medicine has the potential to cause harm as well as benefit, but it is only in the last 10–15 years that efforts to minimize harm have been at the top of the policy agenda. This became a priority in many countries following highly publicized medical disasters that shocked the public and helped to concentrate minds on what could be done to avoid such events in future. In the UK, failures in the performance of surgeons involved in children's heart surgery at Bristol Royal Infirmary between 1984 and 1995 and the subsequent public outcry helped to focus attention on patient safety. The formal inquiry that followed made 198 recommendations on how to prevent such failures (The Bristol Royal Infirmary Inquiry 2001). Among these the inquiry team highlighted the central role of the patient, both as a victim of medical errors and as part of the safety solution.

Patient safety is usually defined in a negative sense as the absence of error or injury. For example, in the USA the influential Institute of Medicine report, *To Err is Human,* defined patient safety as: 'the freedom from accidental injury due to medical care or from medical errors' (Institute of Medicine 2000: 4). This report, and its UK counterpart, *An Organisation with a Memory* (Department of Health 2000), caused considerable concern. What shocked people was the realization that medical errors were quite common, even in what were perceived as the best-performing hospitals. It was estimated that on average one in ten patients admitted to hospital in developed countries were victims of medical errors, and at least half of these could have been prevented.

Medical care is inherently risky and harm can result if mistakes are made in any of a number of routine procedures (Jha et al. 2010). Harm can result from errors of commission (unintentionally doing the wrong thing) or omission (unintentionally not doing the right thing). These can include the following:

- misdiagnosis
- failure to follow up on test results
- unsafe injection practices
- injuries from incorrect use of medical devices
- errors in prescribing medication
- errors in administering medication
- failures in surgical procedures
- wrong-site surgery
- healthcare-associated infections
- falls
- pressure sores
- unsafe blood products
- errors in maternity and neonatal care
- failure to protect children, frail or elderly people.

Both the USA and the UK safety reports concluded that failures such as these are often due not simply to the isolated actions of individuals, but to the way in which health professionals work together and the design of the complex systems in which they work. Many harms or adverse events are the result of a chain of events in which human error plays only a part. Latent failures within healthcare systems create circumstances in which individuals are more prone to error. Instead of blaming individual perpetrators, they argued, what was needed was to design safety features into the systems and processes to reduce the likelihood of errors occurring. They also pointed to the need to build an organizational culture of safety, in which mistakes or service failures could be reported and discussed so that people could analyse the causes, learn from these, and avoid repeating them.

Patients' contribution

Central to the recommendations of the Bristol Inquiry was a belief that enhancing the patient's role (or parent's role in the case of children) could help to prevent the occurrence of errors and harms (Coulter 2002). The report urged doctors to:

- involve patients (or their parents or carers) in decisions
- keep patients and carers informed
- improve communications with patients and carers
- provide patients and carers with counselling and support
- gain informed consent for all procedures and processes
- elicit feedback from patients and carers and listen to their views
- be open and candid when harms or adverse events occur.

Despite this recognition of patients' potential contribution to the avoidance of harm and promotion of safety, there have been few good studies on the impact of involving them. Until recently, their role was almost completely ignored in safety policy, apart from suggestions on how to respond to victims of medical errors and safety risks after they have occurred (Vincent and Coulter 2002). This was despite the fact that many patient and carer groups had played a key role in drawing attention to safety failures and harm done to patients. For example, the Bristol Heart Children Action Group campaigned for the formal inquiry that was eventually set up to investigate what happened at the Bristol Royal Infirmary, leading to a major overhaul of safety procedures throughout the NHS (The Bristol Royal Infirmary Inquiry 2001). Ten years later a group called Cure the NHS was set up by people whose relatives had died or who were themselves victims of poor care at Mid Staffordshire Hospitals Foundation Trust. Their evidence formed an important part of the inquiry into safety failures at the trust which eventually led to government action to strengthen safety procedures (Mid Staffordshire NHS Foundation Trust Inquiry 2010).

In spite of the attention that was paid to their perspective in the official inquiries, many patients and carers felt frustrated and angry that their views were being ignored by NHS organizations. This concern was reflected in a review of the progress of the various patient safety initiatives for the Department of Health in England (Carruthers and Philip 2006: 30). The report included the following comment:

> Consumers of healthcare are at the heart of patient safety. When things go wrong, they and their families suffer from the harm caused. Such harm is often made worse by the defensive and secretive way that many healthcare organisations respond in the aftermath of a serious event.

> Around the world, healthcare organisations that are most successful in improving patient safety are those that encourage close cooperation with patients and their families. Patients and their families have a unique perspective on their experience of healthcare and may provide information and insights that healthcare workers may not otherwise have known.

> Partnership must be a key theme: patients, health professionals, policymakers and healthcare leaders should be working together to prevent avoidable harm in healthcare. A particular focus is to challenge the current culture of denial.

So patients are not just victims of medical errors; they also have much to contribute to improve safety. Various ways in which patients can be involved have been suggested (Coulter and Ellins 2006):

- choosing a safe healthcare provider
- helping to reach an accurate diagnosis
- participating in treatment decision-making
- contributing to safe medication use
- participating in infection control initiatives

- checking the accuracy of medical records
- observing and checking care processes
- identifying and reporting treatment complications and adverse events
- practising effective self-care and monitoring treatments
- providing feedback and advocacy to focus attention on safety issues.

It is helpful to consider each of these issues to understand how the patient's role 'at the heart of patient safety' can be strengthened and supported.

Choosing a safe healthcare provider

Most people know that healthcare involves risks as well as benefits and aware-ness of the potential for harm is growing. A Eurobarometer survey asked res-idents of each of the European Union's 27 member states for their views on the likelihood of harm resulting from medical treatment and whether they had experienced a medical error. Half of all respondents said they felt it was fairly or very likely that they could be harmed while in hospital, ranging from 83 per cent in Greece to only 19 per cent in Austria (TNS Opinion and Social 2010). UK respondents fell somewhere in the middle, with 47 per cent indicating that they were concerned about harm in hospital. The most likely events were said to be hospital-acquired infections or incorrect, missed or delayed diagnoses. More than a quarter said that they or a member of their family had experienced an adverse event due to healthcare, but less than a third of these were reported.

During many recent high-profile medical scandals, such as those at the Bristol Royal Infirmary and the Mid Staffordshire Foundation Trust, it emerged that individual clinicians and professional bodies were aware of lapses in patient safety long before action was taken to investigate and address them. Had the patients involved known about potential risks to their safety, they might have chosen to go to a different provider. This has led to efforts to collate and publish data on quality and safety on publicly accessible websites to enable people to make informed judgments.

Examples include the Leapfrog Group's online database (www. leapfrog-group.org) in the USA and NHS Choices (www.nhs.uk) in the UK. Leapfrog's website includes data on survival rates following surgery and adherence to clinical guidelines derived from survey data. NHS Choices includes data from independent assessments by the Care Quality Commission, including the re-sults of national patient surveys, infection rates reported by hospitals, and survival rates after certain surgical procedures.

However, there is little evidence that publishing performance data improves safety and as yet most patients do not make use of these data when choosing providers (Fung et al. 2008). Most people are unaware of the existence of this performance information, and of those that are, many do not understand the data, do not trust it, or do not view it as useful (Werner and Asch 2005). The same goes for GPs, who tend to rely on informal information sources when making referral decisions, just as patients do (Dixon et al. 2010). Various suggestions have been made for improving the presentation of the data to make it more comprehensible, accessible and useful. It is possible that as patients become more aware of variations in safety indicators they will start acting more like informed, discerning consumers, but at present the performance information that is currently available appears to have had little effect on their choices.

Helping to reach an accurate diagnosis

The information that patients provide to doctors – about their symptoms, concerns and medical and treatment history – is important in establishing early and accurate diagnosis. As with all types of medical error, poor communication and the misunderstandings that can arise from this are a major cause of error in diagnosis. Failure to listen to what the patient is saying about their symptoms, or dismissing their concerns too hastily can lead to misdiagnosis.

A patient-centred consulting style increases the likelihood that important information will be shared (Mead and Bower 2002). For most patients this means a sympathetic doctor who listens and encourages them to discuss their problems (Britten et al. 2000). Barriers to effective communication include clinicians' and patients' interpersonal skills and attitudes, and organizational factors such as the time available for consultations. The effort to overcome these barriers is worth while, because there is increasing evidence that a patient-centred approach can lead to improved patient experience and better health outcomes, including lower mortality rates (Meterko et al. 2010). Patients are more likely than clinicians to view poor communication as a safety problem, with the potential to cause diagnostic delay, physical and psychological harm (Kuzel et al. 2004).

Misunderstandings are quite common in clinician–patient relations, especially if one or both parties finds it difficult to communicate clearly for one reason or another; for example, if they have low proficiency in English, low health literacy, a learning disability or a physical disability. Studies in the USA and Canada have shown that communication problems increase both the risk of preventable adverse events and the likelihood that these will result in physical harm (Bartlett et al. 2008; Divi et al. 2007). Efforts to improve clinician–patient communications should be a central component of initiatives to improve patient safety.

Participating in treatment decision-making

As discussed in Chapter 4, when deciding on the best way to treat or manage a condition, the aim is to maximize the likelihood of desired health outcomes and minimize the chance of undesired consequences. When there is more than one possible course of action, it is important that the patient is informed about the potential benefits and harms of each option and that their values and preferences guide the decision. They cannot be said to have given their informed consent if they have not been fully informed about the risks and involved in the decision. Wennberg has argued that operating on the wrong patient, that is one who would not have wanted the operation if they had been fully informed, is a serious medical error (Wennberg 2010).

There is evidence that patients who are fully aware of the risks of surgical procedures are less likely to want to undergo them than those who are not fully informed (O'Connor et al. 2009). Patients are often more risk-averse than the clinicians who advise them. Evidence from the USA suggests that the states with the highest levels of spending on healthcare, and hence the highest intervention rates, tend to perform worse in terms of quality of care (Baicker and Chandra 2004). Failure to involve and inform patients can lead to over-treatment, which is equivalent to exposing them to unnecessary risk and should therefore be seen as a safety issue.

Contributing to safe medication use

Medication errors are a leading cause of adverse events in healthcare. In the USA it has been estimated that medication errors account for nearly 20 per cent of all incidents that endanger patient safety (Institute of Medicine 2000). Between 1 and 2 per cent of inpatients have been found to have experienced a medication error in both the USA and the UK (Dean et al. 2002). One hundred cases of serious harm from medication errors were reported to the NPSA in 2007 (National Patient Safety Agency 2009b). Of these, 41 per cent were due to errors in administration and 42 per cent to prescribing errors. Elderly people are especially likely to be victims of medication errors because they take more medicines. A study of use of medicines in care homes found that a staggering 70 per cent of residents had experienced a medication error (Barber et al. 2009). Contributing factors included doctors who were not accessible, did not know the residents, and lacked information when prescribing; the high workload of care staff and their lack of medicines training; poor coordination between care staff, GPs and pharmacy; inefficient ordering systems; inaccurate medicine records; and difficult to fill (and check) medication administration systems.

Implementing strategies to reduce the occurrence of preventable medication errors is, therefore, a major element of patient safety initiatives. Patients can contribute to such strategies if they are kept informed about their medicines, including what they are, how they are supposed to work, the reasons for prescribing them, the correct dosage, how to take them, and any likely side-effects. They can be encouraged to speak up if they notice changes in the way they are given or respond to their medicines (Koutantji et al. 2005). Unfortunately patients are not always provided with the information they need. For example, in 2009 45 per cent of patients discharged from hospitals in England said they were not given information about possible side-effects of their medicines (Care Quality Commission 2010).

Patients usually play a central role in the administration of their medicines. To do this effectively they need clear, comprehensible information, well-designed packaging, and an easy way to remember which pill to take when. The standard leaflets in pill packets leave a lot to be desired in terms of useful information (Raynor et al. 2007). There is evidence that improving the packaging can make a difference to patients' ability to remember when and how to take their medicines (Heneghan et al. 2006). Complex interventions, including a combination of information, reminders, follow-up and self-monitoring, can be helpful in improving patients' adherence to prescribed medicines leading to reduced risks and improved outcomes (Haynes et al. 2008).

Participating in infection control initiatives

Infections acquired in hospitals and other healthcare settings are a major patient safety problem. In addition to causing substantial morbidity and mortality, they also prolong hospital lengths of stay, increase resource use, and drive up costs. The main infections that affect hospital patients in England are meticillin-resistant *Staphylococcus aureus* (MRSA) and *Clostridium difficile* (*C. difficile*). They are caused by a wide variety of microorganisms, often by bacteria that normally live harmlessly in or on people's bodies. Scrupulous environmental cleaning, hand washing using soap and alcohol gels, pre-admission screening, isolation of infected individuals, appropriate prescribing of antibiotics and effective wound control are the main means of controlling these infections (Department of Health 2008). While people are most likely to acquire healthcare associated infections during treatment in acute hospitals, they can also occur in GP surgeries, care homes, mental health trusts, ambulances and people's own homes. Around 3 per cent of the public, rising to 6–7 per cent of those admitted to hospital, are carriers of MRSA and C. difficile is present in the gut of about 3 per cent of adults and 66 per cent of infants.

A common source of transmission is direct contact with an infected person, or touching something they have touched. Although not all infections can be prevented, it is estimated that around 50 per cent of cases can be avoided through hand hygiene practices. Patients can encourage compliance with hand hygiene by asking staff who are treating them if they have washed their hands beforehand. The National Patient Safety Agency's *cleanyourhands* campaign assures patients that 'it's ok to ask' healthcare workers to clean their hands before and after they are touched. There is evidence that some patients are willing to take on this role and when they do so it has a beneficial effect (McGuckin et al. 2001; McGuckin et al. 2004). However, many others are reluctant to challenge staff in this way lest it should cause offence.

Cleanliness of hospitals is frequently cited as one of patients' top priorities and fear of hospital associated infections is widespread (Boyd 2007). Patients can be acute observers of hospital procedures, including cleanliness. The national inpatient surveys in England have shown an increasing trend over recent years in the proportion of respondents who said they had observed doctors and nurses always cleaning their hands between touching patients (Picker Institute Europe 2010) (Figure 6.1). However, in 2009 17 per cent said they saw doctors do this only 'sometimes' (18 per cent for nurses) and 7 per cent said they never saw doctors clean their hands (4 per cent for nurses).

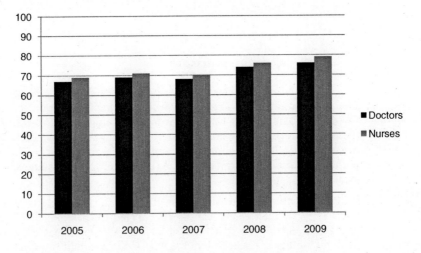

Source: NHS patient survey programme, Care Quality Commission

Figure 6.1 Staff always washed or cleaned their hands between touching patients

Of course, the doctors and nurses may have cleaned their hands out of the patients' line of site. The point is that perceptions of cleanliness and hygiene are important to patients, so it is important to provide reassurance that this basic safety procedure has been complied with.

Checking the accuracy of medical records

Until recently medical records were seen as the property of the clinician rather than the patient. Few patients saw their notes and those that asked to do so were often actively discouraged or reprimanded. Attitudes are slowly changing, but patient-held records are still a rarity.

While there are many enthusiastic advocates for giving patients access to their records and there is evidence that it is feasible, acceptable and useful to both patients and professionals, evidence of the likely effect on patient safety is sparse (Gysels et al. 2007). However, holding their records and reading them can increase patients' knowledge of their health state and their sense of shared responsibility for their own healthcare (see Chapter 4). It can also help to increase the accuracy of the records. One British general practice discovered errors in more than 30 per cent of medical records when patients were encouraged to review their notes (Pyper et al. 2004).

Accurate records are a prerequisite for safe care, so encouraging patients to review them and correct inaccuracies would seem sensible, in addition to the other benefits that this policy can confer.

Observing and checking care processes

Patients can be asked to check the details of their treatment as a safety measure. It is common for staff to ask patients their name and address to reduce the risk of administering a treatment to the wrong person. Unfortunately, the reason for this information check is not always clearly explained to patients, who can be left feeling confused about why they are repeatedly asked to provide the same information. The reasons for this procedure should be explained.

Patients can also be asked to confirm the surgical site (e.g. left leg or right leg?). They, or their carers, can be encouraged to speak up if they notice changes in medication type or dose, or if they suspect that equipment is malfunctioning, or if a bed-bound or chair-bound patient is not moved sufficiently often to prevent bed sores. But challenging staff in this way can prove daunting for patients.

If patients or their relatives are well informed about what ought to happen in respect of clinical procedures, they can draw attention to lapses when they occur (Unruh and Pratt 2007). While patients tend to agree in theory that they could have an important role in monitoring care processes to detect and prevent errors, many are reluctant to do so in practice (Hibbard et al. 2005; Schwappach 2009; Waterman et al. 2006). Strengthening the patient's role will require more than exhortation. They will need better information about what to expect in terms of treatment procedures and active encouragement to monitor and challenge.

The patient's potential role in promoting their own safety is the subject of some debate, however. Many organizations have published advisory leaflets telling patients what they can do to avoid being harmed by inadequate care. Action Against Medical Accidents's (AVMA) suggested tips on how to protect yourself and your family is a typical example:

- Fully discuss the risks involved in any proposed treatment, and any alternatives with your doctor, or other health professional treating you.

- Ask your doctor (or treating health professional) how experienced and successful they are at the treatment (especially surgery) being considered.
- Do not be afraid to ask anyone treating you whether they have washed their hands.
- Just in case something does go wrong, ensure that your household insurance covers you for legal expenses to investigate potential clinical negligence claims.

While this advice seems sensible, some advisories have been criticized on the grounds that they suggest that responsibility for safety can be shifted onto patients (Entwistle et al. 2005). Advice that involves checking on or challenging health professionals' actions may be particularly problematic, especially since there is very little hard evidence that it can be effective (Hall et al. 2010). Instead of burdening the patient with this responsibility, it has been suggested that encouraging patients to observe and challenge should function only as a last resort, with the main responsibility for safety remaining in the hands of health professionals (Davis et al. 2007).

Reporting adverse events

One of the key principles of patient safety policy is that, while it is not always possible to prevent errors and adverse events, much can be learnt from reporting and analysing their occurrence. Many countries have now established incident reporting systems. UK examples include the NPSA's National Reporting and Learning Service (www.npsa.nhs.uk) and the Medicine and Healthcare Products Regulatory Agency's (MHRA) schemes (www.mhra.gov.uk) for reporting adverse drug reactions, incidents relating to the use of medical devices, and problems with blood products or counterfeit medicines and devices. Clinicians and pharmacists are asked to report problems using standardized forms and procedures specially designed for this purpose.

Patients and carers can report problems directly to the clinicians involved in their care, but they are also encouraged to report medicine side-effects or problems with faulty equipment directly to the MHRA. The NPSA also encourages patients to report safety incidents to them directly. When encouraged to do so, patients often report incidents that are not recorded in hospital incident reporting systems (Weingart et al. 2005). Patients' reports of problems with medicines and subsequent campaigns have been instrumental in drawing attention to serious side-effects that were ignored or covered up by pharmaceutical companies. Many patients are concerned about the effects of antidepressant drugs and side-effects are reported quite frequently (van Grootheest et al. 2005). For example, a sustained campaign by Social Audit exposed serious problems with antidepressants such as paroxetine, that had previously been unknown to the public (Medawar and Hardon 2004). There is some evidence that patients report suspected problems with medicines earlier than health professionals, suggesting that patient involvement may help to reduce the time taken to identify and respond to safety issues (Egberts et al. 1996).

Practising effective self-care

As we saw in Chapter 5, patients have a significant role to play in managing their own care. There is evidence that both the quality and outcomes can be enhanced by motivating, equipping and supporting patients in self-management. In the case of those with chronic illnesses, effective self-management is not only desirable but essential.

Patients can contribute to the safe delivery of care through their own active and informed involvement. Patient self-monitoring of anticoagulation therapy, for example, is associated with a reduction in the incidence of serious complications and adverse outcomes (Garcia-Alamino et al. 2010). But they require help to look after themselves effectively, and this is not always forthcoming. For example, among patients discharged from NHS hospitals in 2009, 40 per cent were not told about danger signals to watch out for, 37 per cent were not given any written information about what they should or should not do to promote their recovery, and 33 per cent said no information was given to family members to help them provide after care (Picker Institute Europe 2010).

Advocacy and feedback

A number of advocacy organizations have been set up in recent years to promote the notion that patients have a legitimate right to be involved in patient safety issues. Pre-eminent among these is Patients for Patient Safety, a WHO-sponsored group established in 2004. Their network of patient champions includes members from 50 countries around the world who help to organize campaigns on relevant issues, including hand hygiene and safer surgery through the use of checklists. Other prominent organizations devoted to fostering the patient's role in patient safety include the Action Against Medical Accidents in the UK, the International Alliance of Patients Organizations, a worldwide umbrella group, Consumers Advancing Patient Safety based in Chicago, and the National Patient Safety Foundation based in Boston.

Each of these organizations includes members who have been affected by patient safety issues, often because either they, or their relatives or friends have been victims of medical errors. This gives them a powerful role in explaining to people the causes and consequences of patient safety problems, humanizing what might otherwise be dry statistical accounts. Many are very effective campaigners with a long history of fighting to draw attention to preventable problems and several successes under their belts.

For most patients, however, an easier way to monitor their care and draw attention to any problems is required. Surveys of patients at, or soon after, discharge from hospital, or after an episode of outpatient or primary care can be a useful way to monitor safety issues. Questionnaires have been developed specifically to obtain patients' reports on errors and adverse events (Schwappach 2008). However, most people believe that medical care is fairly safe (Blendon et al. 2002). To avoid alarming them by focusing only on risks, errors and mistakes, it is usually better to include questions about safety in more general patient experience surveys. For example, the national patient surveys in England ask about cleanliness of facilities, observations of hand washing, information about medicines, and so on.

While patient surveys can provide useful indicators of possible safety problems, their reliability will depend on respondents' awareness of the potential for problems and the extent to which staff are open with them. In 2008 the Commonwealth Fund included several questions about medical errors in its regular survey of people with long-term conditions or serious medical events (Schoen et al. 2009). These included whether they had been given the wrong medication or dose in the previous two years, whether any other mistake had been made in their treatment, whether they had been given incorrect lab test results, and whether abnormal test results had been delayed or not provided at all (Figure 6.2).

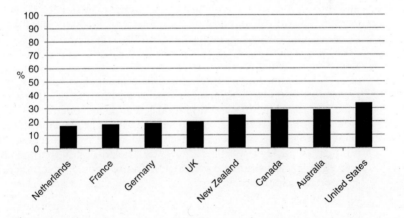

Source: Reproduced from Schoen et al (2009) by permission of the Commonwealth Fund

Figure 6.2 Patients' reported experience of medical errors in eight countries

Respondents from the USA reported twice as many problems as those in the Netherlands. It is impossible to know whether this reflects a greater likelihood of experiencing a medical error in the USA, or whether it is simply the result of greater awareness there of safety problems. Whatever the truth of this international comparison, it is clear that these patients with complex problems had a fairly high likelihood of experiencing a safety problem whichever country they were in. Patients' reports of safety problems have been found to be generally reliable (King et al. 2010), so this is a worrying result.

When things go wrong

If patients are to play a role in ensuring the delivery of safer healthcare, safety improvement programmes must be informed by, and take account of, patients' experience and preferences. Many surveys have shown that patients want more openness about, and disclosure of, medical errors (Burroughs et al. 2007; Evans et al. 2006; Hobgood et al. 2002; Northcott et al. 2008). A British survey of patients who had been affected by medical injury asked about what they wanted and found the following (Chief Medical Officer 2003):

- 34 per cent wanted an apology or explanation
- 23 per cent wanted an enquiry into the causes
- 17 per cent wanted support in coping with the consequences
- 11 per cent wanted financial compensation
- 6 per cent wanted disciplinary action.

Medical injuries can be harder to cope with than other accidents, both because people have been harmed unintentionally by professionals in whom they placed their trust, and because they often have to depend on those same people for further care (Vincent and Coulter 2002). For too many people, the injury is compounded by further trauma due to the insensitive way in which the incident is handled afterwards. When medical errors occur, patients seek not only to be told about the incident but also to receive information on what happened, why it happened, how its consequences can be mitigated and how recurrences can be prevented. Honest disclosure of such information has been found to increase patient satisfaction and trust, and may reduce the likelihood of legal action being commenced (Kachalia et al. 2010). Patients who have been harmed should be treated with empathy and understanding and given appropriate practical and, if necessary, financial help as quickly as possible afterwards. The possibility that the physical injury may be followed by psychological trauma should be considered, and appropriate help provided.

There is, unfortunately, a disparity between patients' preferences for being told about medical mistakes and what happens currently. Patients are frequently not told when medical errors have occurred. Most doctors agree that harmful errors should be disclosed, but they may find it difficult to give full explanations, partly because it can be inherently upsetting and partly because of concerns about legal liability. Both patients and doctors are much more equivocal when it comes to the disclosure of 'near misses', with some patients wanting to know about these but most doctors deeming it inappropriate and unnecessary (Gallagher et al. 2003).

While the case for open disclosure is now widely accepted, it is often poorly implemented (Iedema et al. 2008). Patients and family members complain that explanations are not given promptly enough or only informally; that disclosure is sometimes not followed up with tangible support or a commitment to change practice; and occasionally no apology is offered and patients or relatives are not given an opportunity to meet with the staff involved.

It is clearly important to maintain trust and avoid alarming people unnecessarily, but openness is also very important. This point was reinforced in the National Patient Safety Agency's (NPSA) 'Being Open' policy which stressed the following points (National Patient Safety Agency 2009a):

Being open involves:

- acknowledging, apologizing and explaining when things go wrong
- conducting a thorough investigation into the incident and reassuring patients, their families and carers that lessons learned will help prevent the incident recurring
- providing support for those involved to cope with the physical and psychological consequences of what happened.

The NPSA report also stated that saying sorry is not an admission of liability and is the right thing to do – patients have a right to expect openness in their healthcare and an apology when mistakes have occurred.

Summary

Across the spectrum of patient care there are opportunities for patients to take a role in improving safety and minimizing risk and error. The drive for greater patient involvement must work alongside and complement efforts targeted at the actions of health professionals and system-level vulnerabilities. Patients can be encouraged to raise concerns about safety issues, draw attention to risks and adverse events, provide diagnostic information and participate in treatment decisions. However, genuine forms of patient involvement will only be achieved with a safety culture that appreciates the value of patient contributions and is supportive of these. A culture of this kind will be developed by promoting the principles of openness and honesty, and by encouraging trust and communication between clinicians and patients. As part of this effort, improvements are needed in the way that health professionals share important safety-related information with their patients. This includes committing to full disclosure of medical errors and supporting people who have suffered harm.

References

Baicker, K. and Chandra, A. (2004) Medicare spending, the physician workforce, and beneficiaries' quality of care, *Health Affairs (Millwood)*, Suppl. Web Exclusives: W4–97.
Barber, N.D., Alldred, D.P., Raynor, D.K., Dickinson, R., Garfield, S., Jesson, B., Lim, R., Savage, I., Standage, C., Buckle, P., Carpenter, J., Franklin, B., Woloshynowych, M. and Zermansky, A.G. (2009) Care homes' use of medicines study: prevalence,

causes and potential harm of medication errors in care homes for older people, *Quality and Safety in Health Care*, 18(5): 341–46.

Bartlett, G., Blais, R., Tamblyn, R., Clermont, R.J. and MacGibbon, B. (2008) Impact of patient communication problems on the risk of preventable adverse events in acute care settings, *Canadian Medical Association Journal*, 178(12): 1555–62.

Blendon, R.J., DesRoches, C.M., Brodie, M., Benson, J.M., Rosen, A.B., Schneider, E., Altman, D.E., Zapert, K., Herrmann, M.J. and Steffenson, A.E. (2002) Views of practicing physicians and the public on medical errors, *New England Journal of Medicine*, 347(24): 1933–40.

Boyd, J. (2007) *The 2006 Inpatients Importance Study*. Oxford: Picker Institute Europe.

Britten, N., Stevenson, F.A., Barry, C.A., Barber, N. and Bradley, C.P. (2000) Misunderstandings in prescribing decisions in general practice: qualitative study, *British Medical Journal*, 320(7233): 484–88.

Burroughs, T.E., Waterman, A.D., Gallagher, T.H., Waterman, B., Jeffe, D.B., Dunagan, W.C., Garbutt, J., Cohen, M.M., Cira, J. and Fraser, V.J. (2007) Patients' concerns about medical errors during hospitalization, *Joint Commission Journal on Quality and Patient Safety*, 33(1): 5–14.

Care Quality Commission (2010) *Inpatient Survey 2009*. Newcastle: Care Quality Commission.

Carruthers, I. and Philip, P. (2006) *Safety First: A Report for Patients, Clinicians and Healthcare Managers*. London: Department of Health.

Chief Medical Officer (2003) *Making Amends. A Consultation Paper Setting Out Proposals for Reforming the Approach to Clinical Negligence in the NHS*. London: Department of Health.

Coulter, A. (2002) After Bristol: putting patients at the centre, *Quality and Safety in Health Care*, 11(2): 186–88.

Coulter, A. and Ellins, J. (2006) *Patient-focused Interventions: A Review of the Evidence*. London: The Health Foundation.

Davis, R.E., Jacklin, R., Sevdalis, N. and Vincent, C.A. (2007) Patient involvement in patient safety: what factors influence patient participation and engagement?, *Health Expectations*, 10(3): 259–67.

Dean, B., Schachter, M., Vincent, C. and Barber, N. (2002) Causes of prescribing errors in hospital inpatients: a prospective study, *The Lancet*, 359(9315): 1373–78.

Department of Health (2000) *An Organisation with a Memory: Report of an Expert Group on Learning from Adverse Events in the NHS*. London: The Stationery Office.

Department of Health (2008) *Clean, Safe Care: Reducing Infections and Saving Lives*. London: Department of Health.

Divi, C., Koss, R.G., Schmaltz, S.P. and Loeb, J.M. (2007) Language proficiency and adverse events in US hospitals: a pilot study, *International Journal of Quality Health Care*, 19(2): 60–67.

Dixon, A., Robertson, R., Appleby, J., Burge, P., Devlin, N. and Magee, H. (2010) *Patient Choice: How Patients Choose and How Providers Respond*. London: The King's Fund.

Egberts, T.C., Smulders, M., de Koning, F.H., Meyboom, R.H. and Leufkens, H.G. (1996) Can adverse drug reactions be detected earlier? A comparison of reports by patients and professionals, *British Medical Journal*, 313(7056): 530–31.

Entwistle, V.A., Mello, M.M. and Brennan, T.A. (2005) Advising patients about patient safety: current initiatives risk shifting responsibility, *Joint Commission Journal an Quality and Patient Safety*, 31(9): 483–94.

Evans, S.M., Berry, J.G., Smith, B.J. and Esterman, A.J. (2006) Consumer perceptions of safety in hospitals, *BMC Public Health*, 6: 41.

Fung, C.H., Lim, Y.W., Mattke, S., Damberg, C. and Shekelle, P.G. (2008) Systematic review: the evidence that publishing patient care performance data improves quality of care, *Annals of Internal Medicine*, 148(2): 111–23.

Gallagher, T.H., Waterman, A.D., Ebers, A.G., Fraser, V.J. and Levinson, W. (2003) Patients' and physicians' attitudes regarding the disclosure of medical errors, *Journal of the American Association*, 289(8): 1001–07.

Garcia-Alamino, J.M., Ward, A.M., Alonso-Coello, P., Perrera, R., Bankhead, C., Fitzmaurice, D. and Heneghan, C.J. (2010) Self-monitoring and self-management of oral anticoagulation. *Cochrane Database of Systematic Review*, no. 4.

Gysels, M., Richardson, A. and Higginson, I.J. (2007) Does the patient-held record improve continuity and related outcomes in cancer care: a systematic review, *Health Expectations*, 10(1): 75–91.

Hall, J., Peat, M., Birks, Y., Golder, S., Entwistle, V., Gilbody, S., Mansell, P., McCaughan, D., Sheldon, T., Watt, I., Williams, B. and Wright, J. (2010) Effectiveness of interventions designed to promote patient involvement to enhance safety: a systematic review, *Quality and Safety in Health Care*, 19(5): e.10.

Haynes, R.B., Ackloo, E., Sahota, N., McDonald, H.P. and Yao, X. (2008) Interventions for enhancing medication adherence, *Cochrane Database of System Review*, no. 2: CD000011.

Heneghan, C.J., Glasziou, P. and Perera, R. (2006) Reminder packaging for improving adherence to self-administered long-term medications, *Cochrane Database of System Review*, no. 1: CD005025.

Hibbard, J.H., Peters, E., Slovic, P. and Tusler, M. (2005) Can patients be part of the solution? Views on their role in preventing medical errors, *Medical Care Research Review*, 62(5): 601–16.

Hobgood, C., Peck, C.R., Gilbert, B., Chappell, K. and Zou, B. (2002) Medical errors – what and when: what do patients want to know?, *Academic Emergency Medicine*, 9(11): 1156–61.

Iedema, R., Sorensen, R., Manias, E., Tuckett, A., Piper, D., Mallock, N., Williams, A. and Jorm, C. (2008) Patients' and family members' experiences of open disclosure following adverse events, *International Journal for Quality in Health Care*, 20(6): 421–32.

Institute of Medicine (2000) *To Err is Human: Building a Safer Health System*. Washington, DC: National Academy Press.

Jha, A.K., Prasopa-Plaizier, N., Larizgoitia, I. and Bates, D.W. (2010) Patient safety research: an overview of the global evidence, *Quality and Safety in Health Care*, 19(1): 42–47.

Kachalia, A., Kaufman, S.R., Boothman, R., Anderson, S., Welch, K., Saint, S. and Rogers, M.A.M. (2010) Liability Claims and Costs Before and After Implementation of a Medical Error Disclosure Program, *Annals of Internal Medicine*, 153(4): 213–21.

King, A., Daniels, J., Lim, J., Cochrane, D.D., Taylor, A. and Ansermino, J.M. (2010) Time to listen: a review of methods to solicit patient reports of adverse events, *Quality and Safety in Health Care*, 19(2): 148–57.

Koutantji, M., Davis, R., Vincent, C. and Coulter A. (2005) The patient's role in patient safety: engaging patients, their representatives, and health professionals, *Clinical Risk*, 11(3): 99–104.

Kuzel, A.J., Woolf, S.H., Gilchrist, V.J., Engel, J.D., LaVeist, T.A., Vincent, C. and Frankel, R.M. (2004) Patient reports of preventable problems and harms in primary health care, *Annals of Family Medicine*, 2(4): 333–40.

McGuckin, M., Taylor, A., Martin, V., Porten, L. and Salcido, R. (2004) Evaluation of a patient education model for increasing hand hygiene compliance in an inpatient rehabilitation unit, *American Journal of Infection Control*, 32(4): 235–38.

McGuckin, M., Waterman, R., Storr, I.J., Bowler, I.C., Ashby, M., Topley, K. and Porten, L. (2001) Evaluation of a patient-empowering hand hygiene programme in the UK, *Journal of Hospital Infection*, 48(3): 222–27.

Mead, N. and Bower, P. (2002) Patient-centred consultations and outcomes in primary care: a review of the literature, *Patient Education and Counseling*, 48(1): 51–61.

Medawar, C. and Hardon, A. (2004) *Medicines Out of Control? Antidepressants and the Conspiracy of Goodwill*. Amsterdam: Aksant Academic.

Meterko, M., Wright, S., Lin, H., Lowy, E. and Cleary, P.D. (2010) Mortality among patients with acute myocardial infarction: the influences of patient-centered care and evidence-based medicine, *Health Services Research*, no. DOI: 10.1111/j.1475-6773.2010.011384.

Mid Staffordshire NHS Foundation Trust Inquiry (2010) *Independent Inquiry into Care Provided by Mid Staffordshire NHS Foundation Trust January 2005–March 2009*. London: The Stationery Office.

National Patient Safety Agency (2009a) *Being Open: Communicating Patient Safety Incidents with Patients, their Families and Carers*. London: NPSA.

National Patient Safety Agency (2009b) *Safety in Doses: Improving the Use of Medicines in the NHS 2007*. London: NPSA.

Northcott, H., Vanderheyden, L., Northcott, J., Adair, C., Brien-Morrison, C., Norton, P. and Cowell, J. (2008) Perceptions of preventable medical errors in Alberta, Canada, *International Journal for Quality in Health Care*, 20(2): 115–22.

O'Connor, A.M., Bennett, C.L., Stacey, D., Barry, M., Col, N.F., Eden, K.B., Entwistle, V.A., Fiset, V., Holmes-Rovner, M., Khangura, S., Llewellyn-Thomas, H. and Rovner, D. (2009) Decision aids for people facing health treatment or screening decisions, *Cochrane Database of Systematic Review*, no. 3: CD001431.

Picker Institute Europe (2010) *National NHS Patient Survey Programme: Survey of Adult Inpatients 2009*. London: Care Quality Commission.

Pyper, C., Amery, J., Watson, M. and Crook, C. (2004) Patients' experiences when accessing their on-line electronic patient records in primary care, *British Journal of General Practice*, 54(498): 38–43.

Raynor, D.K., Blenkinsopp, A., Knapp, P., Grime, J., Nicolson, D.J., Pollock, K., Dorer, G., Gilbody, S., Dickinson, D., Maule, A.J. and Spoor, P. (2007) A systematic review of quantitative and qualitative research on the role and effectiveness of written information available to patients about individual medicines, *Health Technology Assessment*, 11(5): iii, 1–iii160.

Schoen, C., Osborn, R., How, S.K., Doty, M.M. and Peugh, J. (2009) In chronic condition: experiences of patients with complex health care needs, in eight countries, 2008, *Health Affairs (Millwood)*, 28(1): w1–16.

Schwappach, D.L. (2008) 'Against the silence': development and first results of a patient survey to assess experiences of safety-related events in hospital, *BMC Health Servicer Research*, 8: 59.

Schwappach, D.L. (2009) Engaging patients as vigilant partners in safety: a systematic review, *Medical Care Research and Review*, 8: 59.

The Bristol Royal Infirmary Inquiry (2001) *The Inquiry into the Management of Care of Children Receiving Complex Heart Surgery at the Bristol Royal Infirmary*. London: Her Majesty's Stationery Office.

TNS Opinion and Social (2010) *Patient Safety and Quality of Healthcare*. Brussels: European Commission Directorate General for Health and Consumers.

Unruh, K.T. and Pratt, W. (2007) Patients as actors: the patient's role in detecting, preventing, and recovering from medical errors, *International Journal of Medical Informatics*, 76(suppl. 1): S236–S44.

van Grootheest, A.C., Passier, J.L. and van Puijenbroek, E.P. (2005) Direct reporting of side effects by the patient: favourable experience in the first year, *Nederlands Tijdschrift voor Geneeskunde*, 149(10): 529–33.

Vincent, C.A. and Coulter, A. (2002) Patient safety: what about the patient?, *Quality and Safety in Health Care* 11(1): 76–80.

Waterman, A.D., Gallagher, T.H., Garbutt, J., Waterman, B.M., Fraser, V. and Burroughs, T.E. (2006) Brief report: hospitalized patients' attitudes about and participation in error prevention, *Journal of General Internal Medicine* 21(4): 367–70.

Weingart, S.N., Pagovich, O., Sands, D.Z., Li, J.M., Aronson, M.D., Davis,. R.B., Bates, D.W. and Phillips, R.S. (2005) What can hospitalized patients tell us about adverse events? Learning from patient-reported incidents, *Journal of General Internal Medicine*, 20(9): 830–36.

Wennberg, J.E. (2010) *Tracking Medicine: A Researcher's Quest to Understand Health Care*. Oxford: Oxford University Press.

Werner, R.M. and Asch, D.A. (2005) The unintended consequences of publicly reporting quality information, *Journal of the American Association*, 293(10): 1239–244.

Further reading

Hurwitz, B. and Sheikh, A. (2009) *Health Care Errors and Patient Safety*. Oxford: Wiley-Blackwell.

Vincent, C. (2010) *Patient Safety*, 2nd edn. Oxford: Wiley-Blackwell.

7 | **Participating in research**

Overview

In this chapter we look at the various ways in which patients can contribute to research, both as study participants, and as contributors to the research process. These roles include determining research priorities, commissioning and reviewing research, designing studies, recruiting participants, measuring health outcomes, gathering and analysing data, disseminating and using research findings.

The importance of patients' role in research

Most healthcare research would be impossible without the active involvement of patients. Without their willingness to participate, there would be no research into biological processes using human tissue, no clinical trials evaluating the effectiveness of drugs, surgery, other treatments and diagnostic tests, very few epidemiological investigations of the causes and consequences of disease, and almost no health services research looking at the quality and outcomes of care. In addition, patients and members of the public play a central role in funding research, both directly, by giving donations to research charities, and indirectly, as taxpayers. And most importantly they are also beneficiaries of research when it leads to a better understanding of how to treat illness and prolong life.

Given their central role in research, it would seem obvious to view patients and members of the public as a primary audience for research findings. Yet most researchers publish papers that are only intended to be read and understood by other academics or clinical specialists. In publicly funded research, it is usual for academics to populate the committees that determine research priorities and select studies for funding; and academics dominate the publishing process too, editing the journals and reviewing papers that report research findings. In commercially funded research, the interests of the companies and their shareholders is pre-eminent. They organize studies in-house or commission academics to carry out laboratory studies and trials of drugs and devices. For the most part the research process is owned and controlled by the producers of research, with minimal involvement from the users – clinicians, managers and patients – but change is on the horizon and patients are at last beginning to exert their influence.

It has been suggested that the quality and relevance of healthcare research could be improved if patients were involved more actively. Potential advantages include greater participation rates, increased external validity, decreased loss to follow up, and benefits for those individuals who are involved (Viswanathan et al. 2004). The last 20 years have seen some important developments in this regard in the UK. For example, the NHS research and development programme, now led by the National Institute for Health Research, has encouraged patient and public involvement since its inception in 1991. Various stakeholders, including patient representatives, are now involved in determining research priorities and deciding which projects will be funded; researchers are required to show how they plan to involve patients and laypeople in their studies when they apply for funding; and websites have been set up to keep the public informed about ongoing research projects that they might want to join.

Participatory research

Participatory or emancipatory research has a long history. Building on various traditions, including community development, adult education, and the disability rights and women's movements, it was borne out of frustration with traditional forms of research that some people felt represented their experiences in ways that were damaging and disempowering (Beresford 2005; Gray et al. 2000). Public involvement in health research is often defined as 'doing research *with* the public, rather than *to, about,* or *for* the public' (Thompson et al. 2009). Now that it has received official endorsement, the response from researchers has been mixed. While many can see benefits of involving laypeople in their studies, others are ambivalent or opposed, viewing it as another regulatory hurdle that can get in the way of effective research.

Most of the published examples of public or lay involvement in research describe studies that were designed and led by academic researchers, with patients or carers in a subordinate role. But there is another strand of activity known as user-led or user-controlled research in which they are more central. In user-controlled research, patients or service users are supposed to lead the study and control all aspects of it, but there are few published examples of studies that have been carried out entirely by patients or carers without professional input (Oliver et al. 2008; Turner and Beresford 2005). In practice, patient participation in research spans a continuum, ranging from involvement in only one part of the process to conducting and controlling the whole study.

There are various ways in which laypeople can play an important role in research, in addition to the traditional roles mentioned above:

- determining research priorities
- commissioning research

- designing studies
- recruiting participants
- measuring health outcomes
- gathering and analysing data
- disseminating and using research findings.

This chapter looks at each of these roles in turn, describing what patients and laypeople can contribute and looking at what happens when they do.

Determining research priorities

Traditionally medical research was investigator-led, with proposals for funding being judged on scientific merit and with little attention paid to its likely relevance to the provision of healthcare. But the rapid increase in research funding and facilities that occurred in the second half of the twentieth century led to various suggestions for prioritizing research expenditure, especially government funding, according to specific criteria.

The NHS research and development programme, launched in 1991, was the first attempt in Britain to establish a coherent system for determining research priorities systematically (Jones et al. 1995). Right from the beginning efforts were made to include laypeople in the prioritization process alongside professional experts. This was not always easy. People, such as managers and patients, who had little or no knowledge of the concept of scientific uncertainty and no previous experience of crafting researchable propositions, struggled to get to grips with academic terminology. Special efforts had to be made to sample the views of ordinary users, alongside the 'professional' consumers from organized groups who were more able to respond to formal consultations.

Experience gained since those early days has led to more sophisticated ways of engaging patients in determining research priorities. The James Lind Alliance (www.lindalliance.org) is one such example (Petit-Zeman et al. 2010). Named after an eighteenth-century Scottish naval surgeon who organized a pioneering clinical trial for the prevention of scurvy, the Alliance encourages groups of patients and clinicians to work together to identify uncertainties about the effects of treatments with a view to stimulating more and better evaluations. Groups identify questions about treatments for which no definitive answers can be found in the literature and then convene workshops to determine priorities. A systematic process known as nominal group technique is used to produce a rank order of research questions. Initially people select and write down their top 10 priorities independently, chosen from the long list of uncertainties, then the combined list is discussed by workshop participants and ranked again until they reach a consensus on their collective top 10. These are then forwarded to research funding bodies.

When patients are involved in setting research priorities they often place greatest emphasis on 'real world' problems experienced by people with the condition. For example, a group convened by the James Lind Alliance, the British Thoracic Society and Asthma UK to determine research needs in asthma care, ranked uncertainties about treatment side-effects and support for self-management at the top of their list of priorities (Elwyn et al. 2010).

The James Lind Alliance has established a database for recording unanswered questions about treatments. Patients, carers and clinicians are invited to contribute to the Database of Uncertainties about the Effects of Treatments (DUETs – www.library.nhs.uk/DUETs). Examples of the types of uncertainties identified by patients are given in Figure 7.1.

- How safe is it for my baby if I am breastfeeding and taking antidepressant medication?
- Is it safe to have a full body massage following myocardial infarction?
- What treatments are best for insomnia while taking antipsychotic drugs for schizophrenia?
- What are the long-term adverse effects of methotrexate tablets when taken for psoriatic arthritis?
- Will avoiding low-energy-saving light bulbs improve my epilepsy?
- At what age should preventative use of statins be started by those with Type 1 diabetes?
- What is the most effective way of managing asthma with other health problems?

Figure 7.1 Examples of treatment uncertainties identified by patients (DUETs)

Encouraging patients and carers to get involved in determining research priorities has much to commend it, but it is by no means the norm as yet. There is often a mismatch between what gets funded and what patients think is important. For example, focus group discussions with people who had osteoarthritis of the knee and a postal survey of a larger group of such patients found that they saw a need for more research on surgical options, physiotherapy, and education and advice, while the majority of published studies looked at drug treatment (Entwistle et al. 2008). The research agenda is still largely shaped by commercial interests and regulatory requirements, rather than by patients' interests. This is a pity because involving patients can broaden the scope of the research agenda and increase its relevance. For example, patients with asthma and chronic obstructive pulmonary disease (COPD) highlighted the importance of more research into medicine side-effects, co-morbidities, interactions between medications, and psychosocial aspects of these conditions which were not adequately covered by current research programmes (Caron-Flinterman et al. 2005). Research funding bodies do not always recognize the fact that patients and laypeople have an important and legitimate role to play in determining priorities.

Commissioning research

Once research priorities have been determined, researchers must be commissioned to carry out the work. The usual method for doing this involves advertising a call for proposals and encouraging research groups to apply. The competitive process is designed to ensure that the commission goes to those who will do the best job, with the most carefully worked out methodology to address the research question as effectively and efficiently as possible. Proposals are usually sent to peer reviewers who scrutinize them carefully and provide reports for consideration by a commissioning board.

Occasionally members of the public are asked to act as lay reviewers of research protocols. Several of the groups that produce systematic reviews for the Cochrane Collaboration routinely invite patients to help them to ensure the relevance and quality of their reviews. For example, the Cochrane Musculoskeletal Group has built a network of patients, carers and laypeople ('consumers' in Cochrane parlance) who guide research priorities, peer review systematic reviews, and promote and facilitate dissemination of the results (Involve 2009; Shea et al. 2005).

In some cases, patients have been able to change the emphasis of a planned study before it begins to make it more relevant to their concerns and more acceptable to potential participants. A review carried out for Involve, a national advisory group that promotes greater public involvement in research, found several examples where service users had challenged the prior assumptions of researchers, leading to a refocusing of studies (Staley 2009). Examples include studies in which laypeople had persuaded the researchers to change the way they conceptualized a topic away from an emphasis on risk reduction towards one that focused on health promotion and empowerment instead.

Sometimes there is lay involvement on the commissioning board itself. This is a tough call for anyone without research experience, since discussions about research methods are often highly technical. Usually the role of laypeople is restricted to reviewing and commenting on proposals. A review of patient and public involvement in the NHS health technology assessment programme found that methodological discussions dominated the commissioning board's decision-making process and the comments of lay reviewers, and indeed clinical peer reviewers, added little to the judgements on the scientific merit of the proposals (Oliver et al. 2006). However, patients may have more to offer when it comes to reviewing less technical topics, especially studies that focus on patients' experience of care.

Designing studies

Patients can contribute valuable 'real world' experience when studies are being planned. They can help to refine the research question, improve the quality of information for participants, and identify important outcomes. When designing questionnaires for use in large-scale surveys it is often good practice to start by consulting patients or involving them in focus groups to learn more about how they experience a particular health problem. For example, a group of patients worked with researchers to refine the interventions and outcome measures for a study of shared decision-making and risk communication in general practice (Thornton et al. 2003). Their involvement led to a better understanding of patients' information needs and a broadening of the range of outcome measures used in the trial.

Diabetes is another clinical area where patients have made an important contribution to study design. Researchers at Warwick University leading a programme of research into diabetes care have described the help they received from a group of patients with a long experience of diabetes who acted as advisers to the project (Lindenmeyer et al. 2007). The main benefit to the researchers was learning more about how it feels to live with diabetes, and how the patients managed to balance the requirement to self-manage their condition with their desire to live a normal life. In another diabetes study, children, teenagers and their families helped with the development phase of the study, including refinement of the interventions and outcome measures (Lowes et al. 2010). Participants' travel expenses were reimbursed and they received £30 in vouchers for each meeting they attended. Most seemed to enjoy the experience. However, involvement in study design can be a time-consuming and expensive process that usually has to be carried out before funding has been obtained. Without external funding it may be hard to accomplish (Staniszewska et al. 2007).

Patients and laypeople often play a useful role in writing, editing or critiquing plain language summaries of the research used when recruiting participants and obtaining informed consent (Hanley et al. 2001). Descriptions that appear clear and obvious to researchers may be less so to laypeople, so these should always be tested with representatives of the intended recipients. This is an important practical task where laypeople can make a useful contribution.

Several researchers have described how patients and service users have made an impact on the selection of outcome measures. For example, Staley describes a clinical trial of a new psychological therapy in which the researchers intended to use neuropsychological tests to check the effects on people's attention, memory and concentration (Staley 2009). Lay reviewers objected to the use of these tests, calling instead for a more relevant and practical outcome measure. Their objections were heeded and the tests were dropped and replaced with a new measure that asked people to remember items on a shopping list. This was considered more relevant and appropriate to those the intervention was intended to benefit.

Recruiting participants

Researchers often struggle to recruit participants into their studies at the rate and frequency specified in the original study protocol. For example, less than half of those invited to take part in treatment trials for cancer agree to do so (Lara et al. 2001). There are various reasons for this, often related to communication or design failures and not giving adequate consideration to patients' attitudes and beliefs. Those responsible for recruitment do not always know how to broach the topic with potential participants in a way that allays their fears or suspicions, or do not present the reasons for the study or its design in a clear, comprehensible or encouraging manner.

Practical considerations can also be a barrier. Studies that involve a great deal of form-filling for participants, frequent interviews or clinic visits at inconvenient times are likely to find recruitment quite difficult. However, most people recognize that participating in studies is a good thing to do, partly because they believe they may benefit from the extra attention that comes with being a study participant, and partly due to altruistic motives and the desire to help others with the same condition or health problem (Jenkinson et al. 2005).

Experimental studies have found that that some recruitment strategies are more likely to be successful than others (Treweek et al. 2010). For example, 'opt-out' recruitment strategies that assume patients will participate unless they specifically decline to do so are more successful than those where patients are invited to opt-in; open trial designs where patients know which treatment they are receiving are often more appealing than blind trials in which the patient does not know whether they have been given an active treatment or a placebo; and telephone reminders have been shown to be a useful way of encouraging people to join in. However, opt-out strategies are controversial and may not be acceptable to an ethics committee; open trials are considered more prone to bias than those where participants and researchers are blinded; and telephone numbers of potential participants may not always be available.

Involving patients or laypeople in an advisory capacity has proved to be helpful in tackling recruitment difficulties. People with insider knowledge of specific local communities can provide advice on the best way to contact participants, can ensure that recruitment procedures and information are appropriate and sensitive to their needs, and can encourage and motivate their peers to take part, especially important when trying to recruit people from minority ethnic communities (Staley 2009). Involvement of patients' organizations can be particularly helpful in demonstrating the importance, legitimacy or credibility of a study and for encouraging people to take part.

A group of researchers from several UK universities who had designed a trial of alternative treatments for prostate cancer were finding it difficult to recruit sufficient patients to participate, so they decided to use qualitative research methods to investigate the recruitment process (Donovan et al. 2002). The trial aimed to compare three treatments for the condition, radical surgery, radiotherapy and non-interventionist treatment, commonly referred to as watchful waiting. They found that some of the terms used by clinician recruiters to describe the options were misunderstood by patients; for example, 'watchful waiting' was misinterpreted as meaning watching the progression of the disease and waiting for the patient to die. Comprehension was improved by substituting the phrase 'active monitoring'. Patients also had difficulty in grasping the concept of equipoise; in other words, that they were eligible for any of the three treatment options, that the most effective treatment was unknown, and that randomization could provide a plausible way of reaching a decision. The qualitative study provided a new understanding of the patients' perspective on the trial which enabled the researchers to improve the content and delivery of information about the study, resulting in an increase in the number agreeing to participate. The recruitment rate increased from 40 per cent to 70 per cent, a significant improvement.

Measuring health outcomes

While clinical trials often include biomedical markers as outcome measures, these do not provide the most important indicators of effectiveness as far as patients are concerned. Most patients seek treatment for symptoms that affect their physical or emotional functioning and sense of well-being or quality of life. Traditional clinical measures of morbidity based on clinical, radiological and laboratory tests do not address these concerns directly. The recognition that the patient's perspective on care and treatment outcomes should be central to the monitoring and evaluation of healthcare led researchers to seek a way of measuring subjective health status and well-being that could be completed by patients themselves.

Patient-reported outcome measures (PROMs) were developed specifically to measure patients' perceptions of the effectiveness of care. They are standardized validated instruments (question sets) to measure patients' perceptions of their health status (impairment), their functional status (disability) and their health-related quality of life (well-being). There are many such instruments available, some focusing on specific diseases or conditions, while others are designed to obtain a generic measure of health outcome. PROMs are usually applied before and after a course of treatment to measure any changes due to the treatment and to assess whether the outcome is beneficial. As well as the standardized instruments, the questionnaires usually include additional questions about the patient's health status and experience of treatment.

In England, PROMs are now being used throughout the NHS as routine outcome measures for people undergoing elective surgery (Hospital Episode Statistics 2010). The decision to introduce the use of PROMs in the NHS in England to measure patients' perspective on health outcomes was a bold move, the first time that routine outcome measurement by all patients undergoing particular procedures had ever been attempted. There are high hopes that it will enable the NHS to measure its impact on people's health more systematically than ever before and that the results will be used widely:

- to inform patients' treatment choices
- to measure and benchmark the performance of healthcare providers

- to incentivize good practice by linking payment to outcomes
- to enable healthcare professionals to monitor and improve practice (Devlin and Appleby 2010).

Since April 2009, patients awaiting procedures such as hip replacement, knee replacement, groin hernia repair and varicose vein surgery have been asked to complete questionnaires before and after their operations. The questionnaires include standardized disease-specific instruments such as the Oxford hip and knee scores and the Aberdeen varicose vein questionnaire, together with the EQ-5D, a generic measure of health status designed for use with a wide range of conditions.

The EQ-5D covers five dimensions of general health:

1 mobility
2 self-care (washing, dressing)
3 usual activities (work, study, housework, family or leisure activities)
4 pain and discomfort
5 anxiety and depression (EuroQol Group 2010).

Each dimension has three levels: no problems, some problems or severe problems. The respondent is asked to indicate his or her health state by ticking the box against the most appropriate statement in each of the five dimensions. The EQ-5D also includes a visual analogue scale indicating how the respondent rates their current health state. The results can be used as a simple profile or combined into a single index score.

The SF-36 is another widely used, well-validated measure of subjective health status (Jenkinson et al. 1993). It covers the following eight domains:

1 physical functioning (e.g. lifting, climbing, bending, walking, dressing)
2 role – physical (impact of physical functioning on everyday life)
3 bodily pain (magnitude and impact)
4 general health
5 vitality (energy, fatigue)
6 social functioning (e.g. interaction with family and friends)
7 role – emotional (impact of social functioning)
8 mental health (e.g. anxiety, depression, stress, happiness).

While the EQ-5D and the SF-36 cover similar issues and often produce broadly similar results, they were derived from different theoretical traditions, use different scoring systems, and were originally intended for different purposes. They are among a proliferation of standardized measures of health status, including both generic and disease-specific instruments. Choice of instrument must be done carefully to ensure selection of the right measure for a particular purpose (Dawson et al. 2010). Often used alongside clinical indicators and measures of patients' experience, they fill an important gap in the measurement of the impact of symptoms and treatments on social functioning and quality of life (Bream and Black 2009).

While it is relatively straightforward to ask patients to complete simple questionnaires before and after an elective procedure, measuring outcomes for people with long-term conditions is more challenging. In these cases there may be no discrete event around which measurement can be planned and patients may have to complete several questionnaires over a period of time to assess the impact of a management strategy, possibly leading to low response rates due to survey fatigue. Another problem is the need to cover a very wide range of conditions and health problems if a true and complete picture of the effectiveness of healthcare is to be obtained. While it would be much simpler to use a simple generic measure such as the EQ-5D with all patients, generic instruments tend to be less sensitive to variations in health status than measures specifically designed for people with a particular condition. As yet no one has developed a health status measure that is suitable for all conditions and settings.

Gathering and analysing data

While involving patients and other laypeople in study design and monitoring is becoming more common, involving them in data-gathering activities such as interviewing other patients or leading focus groups is rarer. This is not surprising. These are skilled tasks and most professional researchers are expected to undergo a considerable amount of education and training before they are entrusted to carry them out. It takes time to learn about and practice research techniques such as questionnaire design, interviewing strategies, avoidance of bias, facilitation skills, ethical considerations, and so on, and few courses are suitable for complete beginners. However, some proponents of participatory research have argued that laypeople should play a central role in all aspects of research, including data-gathering (Turner and Beresford 2005). Peer interviewers, it is argued, can probe more deeply to obtain richer, more reliable information because research participants are more willing to open up and speak honestly to people who are perceived as being 'just like them'.

People with various physical and mental health problems, parents and other carers, and those with learning difficulties have been employed as peer interviewers in a variety of studies. With training, careful supervision and support they are able to carry out particular research tasks quite successfully. For example, a study of parents' views of child health services for babies in the first year of life engaged parents in all aspects of the research process, including facilitating focus groups and analysing the transcripts (Roche et al. 2005). The parent researchers greatly enjoyed leading the focus groups, although they found it quite challenging. Keeping the tone reassuring, supportive and non-judgemental and ensuring that different views are heard is not straightforward for experienced researchers and it may be even more difficult for those who share the experience that is under discussion.

A similar role was played by cancer patients and carers who acted as co-researchers on a study of patients' and carers' views of cancer research (Wright et al. 2006). The peer researchers required a considerable amount of support, both emotional and financial, and the investigators had some initial difficulties in persuading ethics and research governance committees that involvement of lay volunteers in this role was appropriate. Nevertheless, the lead researchers insisted that the effort was worth while and had a beneficial impact on the study.

Active involvement in data-gathering is not always positive for the peer interviewers themselves or for the study. Staley cites examples where inexperienced interviewers failed to probe effectively or failed to understand what interviewees had said (Staley 2009). Sometimes interviewees did not elaborate on certain points because they assumed the interviewer understood them due to their shared experience. Securing sustained involvement of volunteer researchers can also be difficult. Van Staa and colleagues described a study that aimed to engage teenagers with chronic conditions in a study to evaluate hospital services (van Staa et al. 2010). They concluded that it was just about feasible to involve adolescents in this way, but they struggled to attract many participants and those who got involved did not always stay the course. Furthermore, the interviews they carried out lacked depth and did not yield substantial new insights.

As any researcher knows, the research process can be hard work and sometimes quite stressful. For those with particular vulnerabilities, for example, people with mental health problems or learning difficulties, it may be difficult to achieve sufficient detachment from the subject matter, leading to emotional distress and sometimes harrowing experiences (Clark et al. 2005; Tuffrey-Wijne and Butler 2010). Lay researchers are likely to require a significant amount of close supervision and support. While the individuals themselves may benefit from the experience of working alongside professional researchers, the question remains about whether the extra effort has a significantly beneficial impact on the study to justify it in terms of cost-effectiveness.

Disseminating and using research findings

Many people believe that researchers have a moral obligation to inform study participants about their findings. When invited to express a preference, most participants want to see a summary of the study results, but they frequently do not get an opportunity to do so (Dalal et al. 2009). After the trials and tribulations of organizing a study and getting the results ready for publication, often long after the period of funding has finished, it can be hard to find time for the extra work involved in sending summaries to all those involved in the study. Ethical requirements may get in the way if, for example, names and addresses of participants have been destroyed to preserve anonymity; journal requirements may preclude any publicity prior to publication; and research assistants on short-term contracts may have moved on to other posts before this stage is reached.

When patients are directly involved in the conduct of the study they can provide helpful input at the dissemination stage. Staley cites examples where lay participants have helped to engage the target audience by alerting local agencies; in some cases they have made the findings more accessible and the messages more powerful by presenting the results at meetings and conferences; by endorsing the findings patients can sometimes enhance the credibility of the results by letting healthcare providers 'hear it from the horse's mouth'; and in some cases they have devised novel ways of transmitting the learning, such as the peer researchers in a mental health study who devised a play to transmit the learning to professionals (Staley 2009).

Charities and patients' organizations frequently play an important role in interpreting and summarizing research findings for their members, ensuring that they are presented in a clear and comprehensible manner and widely disseminated. For example, Macmillan Cancer Support produces a wide range of booklets, audiotapes, toolkits and handbooks to inform people with cancer about prognosis and treatments for different types of cancer, derived from research evidence. Their materials are certified by the Department of Health's Information Standard as a guarantee of reliability, and versions are available in Braille and other forms, ensuring they are accessible to people with vision impairment.

Apart from general interest and a desire to see what has resulted from their participation in a study, patients often need specific research information when they are making decisions about their health and care. Websites, such as NHS Choices (www.nhs.uk) are one means of disseminating research evidence to patients, and patient decision aids (see Chapter 4) are another. The mass media is the dissemination vehicle with potentially the greatest reach, although as we have seen (Chapter 3) they cannot always be relied upon to report research accurately. Making use of each of these methods to disseminate research findings is the best way to ensure that these reach members of the public in an accessible and comprehensible form.

Patients sometimes get involved in helping to translate research evidence into practical action through participation in clinical audit programmes. They can potentially play a role in all four stages of the audit cycle – preparation and planning, measuring performance, implementing change and sustaining improvement. Successful involvement requires both patients and clinicians being clear about their respective roles, supported by excellent communications and organizational commitment to patient engagement. Patients have been involved in everything from large national audits covering entire specialties to small audit projects in a single clinic or general practice. The Myocardial Ischaemia National Audit Project (MINAP) is an example of the former, with patients and carers sitting on the steering group, participating in regional roadshows, and helping to ensure that project reports provide useful public information. Patients who get involved in this way are often strong supporters of the programmes. For example, one of the patient members of the MINAP steering group said:

> If MINAP were a new drug it would be hailed as a life-saver. That's exactly what it is doing, helping to save the lives of heart attack patients by encouraging hospitals and ambulance trusts to improve performances.
>
> (Healthcare Quality Improvement Partnership and National Voices 2009: 18)

Supporting involvement in research

Encouraging laypeople to join research projects should not be undertaken lightly. It requires skills, time, training, funding and support. Simply inviting untrained and inexperienced people to join a group of academic researchers and/or health professionals and hoping they will make a difference to the decision-making process is unlikely to be effective. They are likely to find discussions about research protocols and methodologies confusing and may be frustrated, intimidated or bored.

Since it is costly and time-consuming, patient involvement in research is only worth doing if the goals are clear; for example, to improve the quality of the study or give it added credibility making it more likely that the results will be taken note of and acted upon. As well as being clear about the rationale for involvement, careful consideration should be given to several other important issues before recruiting patients to join a study. For example, deciding which aspects of the study they will be involved in and what level of involvement is appropriate; developing a recruitment strategy and a training plan; considering any ethical or methodological issues that may arise during the course of the study and how these will be dealt with; and devising a payment policy, including payment of expenses (Wright et al. 2010).

Building on their collective experience of participatory research, a group of about 100 researchers used formal consensus methods to devise a set of principles for successful consumer involvement in NHS research (Telford et al. 2004) (Figure 7.2).

Applying these principles successfully will require considerable advance planning before launching into a research project and ongoing commitment to involve patients at all stages.

Assessing impact

As experience grows of involving patients and members of the public, understanding of the complexity of the task is becoming clearer. Attention is now turning to questions about whether the effort is worth while and how to assess its impact.

There is still considerable doubt about the added value of lay involvement in research. Patients and carers are often motivated to get involved in research

1 The roles of consumers are agreed between the researchers and consumers involved in the research
2 Researchers budget appropriately for the costs of consumer involvement in research
3 Researchers respect the differing skills, knowledge and experience of consumers
4 Consumers are offered training and personal support to enable them to be involved in the research
5 Researchers ensure that they have the necessary skills to involve consumers in the research process
6 Consumers are involved in decisions about how participants are both recruited and kept informed about the progress of the research
7 Consumer involvement is described in research reports
8 Research findings are available to consumers, in formats and in language they can easily understand.

Source: Reproduced from Telford et al. (2004) with permission from John Wiley & Sons

Figure 7.2 Principles of successful consumer involvement in NHS research

by a desire to improve care and change services for the better. However, it can be difficult to assess the impact of their involvement, either in terms of better quality studies or better services. While there are many anecdotal accounts of beneficial effects, there is very little hard evidence on impact, either positive or negative. Staley mentions several reasons for this (Staley 2009):

- It is often too difficult or too costly to set up a comparison project without involvement to assess the impact of involvement on study quality and outcomes.
- The most valuable contributions from the public come from personal interactions with researchers which are hard to capture and evaluate.
- Patients are often involved in research committees or steering groups but it is extremely difficult to evaluate the impact of any individual on the group's decisions.
- Involvement activities are interconnected and link to several stages of the research process, making it difficult to pinpoint the precise impact of any particular activity.
- It may take many years for any detectable outcomes to emerge from a study.

Summary

Most healthcare research would be impossible without patient participation. Many people have suggested that encouraging patients, carers and other laypeople to get actively involved in the design and conduct of studies could help to improve the quality and relevance of studies and enhance their impact. It is generally agreed that patients can play a valuable role in determining research priorities, in study design, in helping to recruit participants, in measuring health outcomes, and in disseminating the findings. There is more debate about the merits of involving them in commissioning research, or gathering and analysing data, since these are highly technical tasks requiring extensive training and supervision. There is little evidence, as yet, to support claims that patient involvement improves the quality and impact of research.

References

Beresford, P. (2005) Theory and practice of user involvement in research, in L. Lowes and I. Hulatt (eds), *Involving Service Users in Health and Social Care Research* (pp. 6–17). London: Routledge.

Bream, E. and Black, N. (2009) What is the relationship between patients' and clinicians' reports of the outcomes of elective surgery?, *Journal of Health Services Research and Policy*, 14(3): 174–82.

Caron-Flinterman, J.F., Broerse, J.E., Teerling, J. and Bunders, J.F. (2005) Patients' priorities concerning health research: the case of asthma and COPD research in the Netherlands, *Health Expectations*, 8(3): 253–63.

Clark, M., Lester, H. and Glasby, J. (2005) From recruitment to dissemination: the experience of working together from service user and professional perspectives, in L. Lowes and I. Hulatt (eds), *Involving Service Users in Health and Social Care Research* (pp. 76–84). London: Routledge.

Dalal, H., Wingham, J., Pritchard, C., Northey, S., Evans, P., Taylor, R.S. and Campbell, J. (2009) Communicating the results of research: how do participants of a cardiac rehabilitation RCT prefer to be informed?, *Health Expectations*, 13(3): 323–30.

Dawson, J., Doll, H., Fitzpatrick, R., Jenkinson, C. and Carr, A.J. (2010) Routine use of patient reported outcome measures in healthcare settings, *British Medical Journal*, 340, c186.

Devlin, N. and Appleby, J. (2010) *Getting the Most Out of PROMs: Putting Health Outcomes at the Heart of NHS Decision-Making*. London: King's Fund.

Donovan, J., Mills, N., Smith, M., Brindle, L., Jacoby, A., Peters, T., Frankel, S., Neal, D. and Hamdy, F. (2002) Quality improvement report: improving design and conduct of randomised trials by embedding them in qualitative research: ProtecT (prostate testing for cancer and treatment) study. Commentary: presenting unbiased information to patients can be difficult, *British Medical Journal*, 325(7367): 766–70.

Elwyn, G., Crowe, S., Fenton, M., Firkins, L., Versnel, J., Walker, S., Cook, I., Holgate, S., Higgins, B. and Gelder, C. (2010) Identifying and prioritizing uncertainties: patient and clinician engagement in the identification of research questions, *Journal of Evaluation in Clinical Practice*, 16(3): 627–31.

Entwistle, V., Calnan, M. and Dieppe, P. (2008) Consumer involvement in setting the health services research agenda: persistent questions of value, *Journal of Health Services Research and Policy*, 13(Suppl. 3): 76–81.

EuroQol Group (2010) *EQ-5D: A Standardised Instrument for Use as a Measure of Health Outcome*. Available online at www.euroqol.org.

Gray, R.E., Fitch, M., Davis, C. and Phillips, C. (2000) Challenges of participatory research: reflections on a study with breast cancer self-help groups, *Health Expectations*, 3(4): 243–52.

Hanley, B., Truesdale, A., King, A., Elbourne, D. and Chalmers, I. (2001) Involving consumers in designing, conducting, and interpreting randomised controlled trials: questionnaire survey, *British Medical Journal*, 322: 519–23.

Healthcare Quality Improvement Partnership and National Voices (2009) *Patient and Public Engagement in Clinical Audit*. Available online at www.hqip.org.uk/assets/PPE/HQIP-PPE-Guidance.pdf.

Hospital Episode Statistics (2010) *Provisional Monthly Patient Reported Outcome Measures (PROMs) in England: April 2009–April 2010*. London: NHS Information Centre.

Involve (2009) *Senior Investigators and Public Involvement*. Eastleigh: Involve.

Jenkinson, C., Burton, J.S., Cartwright, J., Magee, H., Hall, I., Alcock, C. and Burge, S. (2005) Patient attitudes to clinical trials: development of a questionnaire and results from asthma and cancer patients, *Health Expectations*, 8(3): 244–52.

Jenkinson, C., Coulter, A. and Wright, L. (1993) Short form 36 (SF36) health survey questionnaire: normative data for adults of working age, *British Medical Journal*, 306(6890): 1437–40.

Jones, R., Lamont, T. and Haines, A. (1995) Setting priorities for research and development in the NHS: a case study on the interface between primary and secondary care, *British Medical Journal*, 311(7012): 1076–80.

Lara, P.N., Jr., Higdon, R., Lim, N., Kwan, K., Tanaka, M., Lau, D.H., Wun, T., Welborn, J., Meyers, F.J., Christensen, S., O'Donnell, R., Richman, C., Scudder, S.A., Tuscano, J., Gandara, D.R. and Lam, K.S. (2001) Prospective evaluation of cancer clinical trial accrual patterns: identifying potential barriers to enrollment, *Journal of Clinical Oncology*, 19(6): 1728–33.

Lindenmeyer, A., Hearnshaw, H., Sturt, J., Ormerod, R. and Aitchison, G. (2007) Assessment of the benefits of user involvement in health research from the Warwick Diabetes Care Research User Group: a qualitative case study, *Health Expectations*, 10(3): 268–77.

Lowes, L., Robling, M.R., Bennert, K., Crawley, C., Hambly, H., Hawthorne, K. and Gregory, J.W. (2010) Involving lay and professional stakeholders in the development of a research intervention for the DEPICTED Study, *Health Expectations*, DOI: 10.1111/j.1369-7625.2010.00625.x.

Oliver, S., Armes, D. and Gyte, G. (2006) *Evaluation of Public Influence on the NHS Health Technology Assessment Programme*. London: Social Science Research Unit, Institute of Education, University of London.

Oliver, S.R., Rees, R.W., Clarke-Jones, L., Milne, R., Oakley, A.R., Gabbay, J., Stein, K., Buchanan, P. and Gyte, G. (2008) A multidimensional conceptual framework for analysing public involvement in health services research, *Health Expectations*, 11(1): 72–84.

Petit-Zeman, S., Firkins, L. and Scadding, J.W. (2010) The James Lind Alliance: tackling research mismatches, *The Lancet*, 376(9742): 667–69.

Roche, B., Savile, P., Aikens, D. and Scammell, A. (2005) Consumer led research? Parents as researchers: the child health surveillance project, in L. Lowes and I. Hulatt (eds), *Involving Service Users in Health and Social Care Research* (pp. 85–96). London: Routledge.

Shea, B., Santesso, N., Qualman, A., Heiberg, T., Leong, A., Judd, M., Robinson, V., Wells, G. and Tugwell, P. (2005) Consumer-driven health care: building partnerships in research, *Health Expectations*, 8(4): 352–59.

Staley, K. (2009) *Exploring Impact: Public Involvement in NHS, Public Health and Social Care Research*. Eastleigh: Involve.

Staniszewska, S., Jones, N., Newburn, M. and Marshall, S. (2007) User involvement in the development of a research bid: barriers, enablers and impacts, *Health Expectations*, 10(2): 173–83.

Telford, R., Boote, J.D. and Cooper, C.L. (2004) What does it mean to involve consumers successfully in NHS research? A consensus study, *Health Expectations*, 7(3): 209–20.

Thompson, J., Barber, R., Ward, P.R., Boote, J.D., Cooper, C.L., Armitage, C.J. and Jones, G. (2009) Health researchers attitudes towards public involvement in health research, *Health Expectations*, 12(2): 209–20.

Thornton, H., Edwards, A. and Elwyn, G. (2003) Evolving the multiple roles of 'patients' in health-care research: reflections after involvement in a trial of shared decision-making, *Health Expectations*, 6(3): 189–97.

Treweek, S., Pitkethly, M., Cook, J., Kjeldstrom, M., Taskila, T., Johansen, M., Sullivan, F., Wilson, S., Jackson, C., Jones, R. and Mitchell, E. (2010) Strategies to improve recruitment to randomised controlled trials, *Cochrane Database of Systematic Review*, 4: MR000013.

Tuffrey-Wijne, I. and Butler, G. (2010) Co-researching with people with learning disabilities: an experience of involvement in qualitative data analysis, *Health Expectations*, 13(2): 174–84.

Turner, M. and Beresford, P. (2005) *User Controlled Research: Its Meanings and Potential*. Eastleigh: Involve.

van Staa A., Jedeloo, S., Latour, J.M. and Trappenburg, M.J. (2010) Exciting but exhausting: experiences with participatory research with chronically ill adolescents, *Health Expectations*, 13(1): 95–107.

Viswanathan, M., Ammermam, A., Eng, E., Gartlehner, G., Lohr, K.N., Griffith, D., Rhodes, S., Samuel-Hodge, C., Maty, S., Lux, L., Webb, L., Sutton, S.F., Swinson, T., Jackman, A. and Whitener, L. (2004) *Community Based Participatory Research: Assessing the Evidence*. Agency for Healthcare Research and Quality, Rockville, MD: Evidence Report/Technology Assessment 99.

Wright, D., Corner, J., Hopkinson, J. and Foster, C. (2006) Listening to the views of people affected by cancer about cancer research: an example of participatory research in setting the cancer research agenda, *Health Expectations*, 9(1): 3–12.

Wright, D., Foster, C., Amir, Z., Elliott, J. and Wilson, R. (2010) Critical appraisal guidelines for assessing the quality and impact of user involvement in research, *Health Expectations*, DOI: 10.1111/j.1369-7625.2010.00607.x.

Further reading

Lowes and L. and Hulatt, I. (2005) *Involving Service Users in Health and Social Care Research*. London: Routledge.

Nolan, M., Hanson, E., Grant, G. and Keady, J. (2007) *User Participation in Health and Social Care Research*. Maidenhead: Open University Press.

Staley, K. (2009) *Exploring Impact: Public Involvement in NHS, Public Health and Social Care Research*. Eastleigh: Involve.

8 Training professionals

Overview

This chapter looks at professional training and how it must adapt to meet the changing needs and expectations of patients and new patterns of healthcare delivery. We look at what is being done to meet the new demands and at the standards and learning outcomes that students and trainees are required to achieve. The objectives of communication skills training and barriers to effective communication are discussed. Strategies for improving patients' experience of healthcare, such as interprofessional education and cultural competence training, are briefly reviewed. Finally, we look at the role of patients in professional education, both simulated patients and real patients, and the impact of involving them in teaching.

Educational challenges

The training of health professionals is key to achieving improvements in healthcare quality. In addition to biological knowledge and scientific and technical skills, health professionals must learn how to interact with and care for patients. As we have seen in previous chapters, what patients and the public expect from health professionals is changing. It has always been expected that education for medical, nursing and allied health trainees would equip them with clinical knowledge and practical skills, as well as inculcating a professional culture that emphasizes their responsibility to be trustworthy and act in the best interests of their patients. But nowadays more is expected of them. Patients want clinicians who can empathize and understand what it means to be ill, who listen to them and respect their concerns and preferences, who inform and involve them and support their efforts in self-care. They also want more responsive, better integrated health systems that provide effective, equitable, well coordinated care, plus support for disease prevention and health promotion.

Arthur Kleinman argued that modern medicine was in danger of forgetting part of its central purpose. Clinicians should focus not only on control of disease processes, but also on the experience of illness:

> When viewed from the human situations of chronic illness, neither the interpretation of illness meanings nor the handling of deeply felt emotions within intimate personal relationships can be dismissed as peripheral tasks.

They constitute, rather, the point of medicine. These are the activities with which the practitioner should be engaged. The failure to address these issues is a fundamental flaw in the work of doctoring.

(Kleinman 1988: 253)

He went on to suggest that professional training programmes should make the patient's and the family's narrative of the illness experience more central in the education process. This would require the development of new ways of teaching about clinician–patient relationships with a particular emphasis on caring for people who are chronically ill.

So trainees require at least a basic understanding of psychology, sociology, and other behavioural sciences, together with some knowledge of cultural diversity and the economic, social, and environmental determinants of public health. They must learn about how people experience disease and treatment, and about different cultural attitudes and health beliefs. They must know how to communicate clearly and effectively with patients, and how to support them through illness and recovery. Trainees also need a sound grasp of how health systems work, together with knowledge of community-based sources of support for patients and their families. And they must develop the leadership and teamworking skills necessary to transform health systems.

Future training needs

It takes a long time to train to be a health professional. Basic training for nurses takes three years but many go on to do further training; allied health professionals usually do at least two to three years of postgraduate study plus practical experience; and doctors must train for a minimum of nine years if they want to go into general practice, and for twelve years or more if they want to be a hospital-based specialist. Even so, covering the full range of knowledge and skills required is difficult. A major challenge for those planning these programmes is how to ensure that courses accurately anticipate future developments in healthcare technology and in public expectations. The long training period, coupled with difficulties inherent in developing, agreeing and implementing new curricula, makes it hard to keep up with the rapid pace of change. Courses are often planned many years in advance, requiring curriculum designers to anticipate likely requirements some 15–20 years hence.

An independent commission into the education of health professionals worldwide concluded that professional education has failed to keep up with these challenges (Frenk et al. 2010: 1923). They described the problems in the following terms:

The problems are systemic: mismatch of competencies to patient and population needs; poor teamwork; persistent gender stratification of professional status; narrow technical focus without broader contextual understanding; episodic encounters rather than continuous care; predominant hospital orientation at the expense of primary care; quantitative and qualitative imbalances in the professional labour market, and weak leadership to improve health system performance.

The commission called for major reform of global professional education systems in pursuit of a common vision (Frenk et al. 2010: 1924):

All health professionals in all countries should be educated to mobilise knowledge and to engage in critical reasoning and ethical conduct so that they are competent to participate in patient and population-centred health systems as members of locally responsive and globally connected teams. The ultimate purpose is to assure universal coverage of the high-quality comprehensive services that are essential to advance opportunity for health equity within and between countries.

Various attempts have been made to forecast future training needs. The Royal College of Physicians and Surgeons in Canada concluded that doctors must learn to play several different roles (Royal College of Physicians and Surgeons in Canada 2010):

- collaborator (the ability to work in a team to achieve optimal patient care)
- manager (active participation in a healthcare system with responsibility for contributing to its effectiveness)
- health advocate (promoting the health of patients, communities and populations)
- scholar (committed to lifelong reflective learning as well as contributing to new knowledge and practices)
- professional (committed to ethical practice, profession-led regulation and high standards of personal behaviour).

Similar reviews were organized in England to assess the future training needs of doctors (Postgraduate Medical Education and Training Board 2008) and nurses and midwives (Prime Minister's Commission on the Future of Nursing and Midwifery in England 2010). Between them these reports detailed a number of specific competences that would be required, underscoring the need to teach professionals how to balance their duty to individual patients with those of the wider population (Figure 8.1).

Squeezing all this into already full curricula is a tall order, but unless training programmes take account of these issues they will quickly become out of date and trainees will be ill-prepared to meet patients' needs and expectations. Involving patients and carers in curriculum planning for professional training could help to ensure that patients' needs are kept on the agenda.

Setting standards

Recent years have seen a shift towards competence-based curricula. This includes specification of the competences (learning outcomes) required for patient engagement. In the past, postgraduate medical training took the

Interpersonal knowledge, skills and attitudes
- Understanding the patient's perspective, listening actively, expressing empathy and communicating clearly
- Eliciting and taking account of patients' preferences
- Communicating information on risk and probability
- Sharing treatment decisions
- Providing support for self-care and self-management
- Guiding patients to appropriate sources of information on health and healthcare
- Being aware of alternative sources of support for patients, including those provided by the voluntary sector, and signposting these when appropriate
- Educating patients on how to protect their health and prevent occurrence or recurrence of disease
- Working effectively in multidisciplinary teams while maintaining a focus on the needs of patients
- Learning how to deal with patients' varying needs and expectations and how to negotiate and resolve conflict.

Population-focused knowledge skills and attitudes
- Working across professional boundaries to meet the complex care needs of an ageing population
- Being alert to cultural differences among patient groups and responding to these appropriately
- Being aware of the particular needs of certain sub-groups; for example, those with learning disabilities or mental health problems
- Maintaining generalist skills in the face of a general trend towards greater specialization
- Managing time and resources efficiently
- Using new technologies effectively
- Understanding the principles of patient safety and what to do when things go wrong
- Learning about the factors that impact on public health, how to encourage the adoption of healthier behaviours and how to tackle health inequalities
- Dealing with the requirements of accountability and public scrutiny
- Keeping abreast of relevant research evidence and the principles of evidence-based practice
- Understanding performance and outcomes measurement, quality improvement and quality assurance, including clinical governance and revalidation

Figure 8.1 Competences for modern professional practice

form of an apprenticeship to a 'firm' of doctors, relying on observation of role models and close supervision by seniors. Since the early 1990s, the move to reduce junior doctors' working hours resulted in the gradual abolition of the firm structure. In its place has emerged a more formal educational system that offers trainees less supervised learning time and less consistency in who supervises them, but greater focus on what they must learn and how they are assessed. This required the adoption of specified curricula with defined learning objectives and common assessment standards.

The same developments have affected nurse training. Formerly based on a traditional apprenticeship model, in the 1990s it moved into universities, developed formal curricula, and nurses had to study traditional academic subjects such as sociology and psychology alongside clinical skills. Some people voiced concerns about this shift towards making nursing an all-graduate profession. In particular there were worries that the curriculum was being overloaded with theory, with less time for practical learning. These concerns encouraged the government and regulators to intervene with various policy initiatives designed to increase the emphasis on acquiring specific skills to be learnt and practised in the 'real world' of healthcare facilities (Stark and Stronach 2005).

The General Medical Council (GMC) and the Nursing and Midwifery Council (NMC) are responsible for overseeing the education of doctors and nurses in the UK. They set the standards for good practice and determine the expected outcomes of professional training programmes. Both organizations have recently revised their standards to strengthen the emphasis on patient-centred care. The GMC's document, *Good Medical Practice* and the NMC's *The Code*, describe what is expected of doctors and nurses in similar terms (General Medical Council 2009a; Nursing and Midwifery Council 2008). Both documents emphasize the need to make the care of patients the first concern, treating them as individuals, respecting their dignity and working in partnership with them. Other regulatory bodies, such as the General Pharmaceutical Council and the Health Professions Council, have similar codes of conduct and standards of proficiency (General Pharmaceutical Council 2010; Health Professions Council 2008).

Communication skills and shared decision-making are stressed by both organizations as key competences that must be taught. For example, the GMC states that medical school students must learn how to communicate clearly, sensitively and effectively with patients and their families. This includes those with special needs; for example, people for whom English is not the first language, and those with mental health problems, physical or learning disabilities (General Medical Council 2009b). Trainees must learn how to elicit patients' questions, their understanding of their condition and treatment options, and their concerns and preferences. The NMC states that all nurses must be able to build partnerships and therapeutic relationships through safe, effective and non-discriminatory communication, taking account of individual differences, capabilities and needs (Nursing and Midwifery Council

2010). Nurses should use a range of communication skills and technologies to support person-centred care and they must be ready to provide patients with the information they need to allow them to make informed choices.

Learning to communicate

Since 2002, the ability to communicate competently with patients has been a pre-condition of qualification for all healthcare professionals wanting to work in the NHS. Communication skills are now widely taught in undergraduate and basic professional training courses. Important research has been done to develop understanding of the interpersonal skills that health professionals require, especially in general practice, and this has influenced training programmes. Numerous textbooks have been published on the topic and a wide variety of approaches are advocated. One of the most widely used is the Calgary–Cambridge framework, which divides the consultation into five stages with a list of tasks that must be accomplished in each (Kurtz et al. 2003) (Figure 8.2).

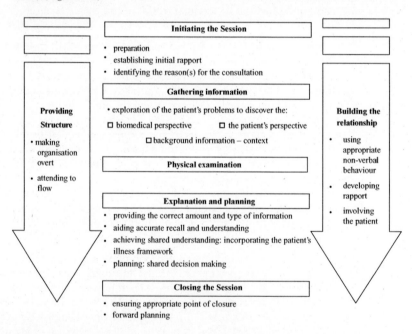

Source: Reproduced from Kurtz et al. (2003) with permission from Wolters Kluwer Health

Figure 8.2 Calgary–Cambridge guide to the medical interview

The problem with the task-based approach is that it assumes that the doctor will control the entire process, leaving little room for the patient to take the discussion down a different track. While this may be a sensible, pragmatic strategy to ensure that the business can be completed within tight time constraints, there is growing interest in searching for alternative, less directive models (Collins et al. 2007).

One problem identified by researchers is a tendency among doctors to avoid discussing the emotional impact of patients' problems, using blocking behaviour to avoid the issue; for example, by attending to the physical aspects only, explaining away distress as normal, or switching topics (Maguire and Pitceathly 2002). The importance of establishing eye contact has been noted, as well as asking about the patient's perceptions and feelings, responding to cues about problems and distress, clarifying and exploring these, and demonstrating interest in the patient's psychosocial well-being.

The good news is that there is evidence that, with effective teaching and ample opportunity to practise, effective interpersonal skills can be learnt and reproduced, resulting in better consultations. For example, trainees can be taught how to express empathy (Bonvicini et al. 2009), how to practise shared decision-making (Bieber et al. 2009), and how to break bad news (Makoul et al. 2010). Well-designed training programmes can increase the patient-centredness of consultations leading to improved patient satisfaction (Gysels et al. 2004; Lewin et al. 2001). There remains a question mark, however, about the extent to which these skills can be sustained when faced with the real world pressures of a busy clinic.

The hidden curriculum

Despite the shift to more formal curricula, role modelling is still an important component of education and training in medicine. Much postgraduate medical education takes place in workplace settings under supervision. Trainees are expected to learn not only the essential clinical knowledge and skills to enable them to do their jobs, but also to absorb and demonstrate appropriate attitudes and ways of behaving towards patients. Their success in this endeavour is likely to be influenced by the 'hidden curriculum', the norms and values they absorb when observing the behaviour of those around them. If they are presented with role models whose interactions with patients are paternalistic or directive, there is a strong likelihood they will forget what they have been taught and instead adopt these observed behaviours.

The dominance of the 'hard' sciences in medicine can sometimes create a lack of sympathy for what is seen as 'soft' evidence, such as the need for empathic communication. In some specialist programmes there is a tendency to encourage trainees to focus on the disease rather than the patient and their social context, downplaying both the complexity of the encounter and the importance of patients' values, preferences and self-knowledge (Corke et al. 2005; Stevenson et al. 2004). The focus on interpersonal relations, which draws on the social sciences for its evidence base, is seen by some clinicians as not truly 'scientific', and hence not a high priority. If this knowledge is not rigorously assessed in the exams that students must pass, it can be viewed as unimportant by medical students. Antipathy to the topic of interpersonal skills on the part of sections of the medical establishment is shared by some students, most of whom gain entry to medical school on the basis of their abilities in the natural sciences rather than the social sciences. New medical graduates often find themselves working in highly pressured environments surrounded by a medical culture that places more value on technical skills than on engaging patients.

Various commentators have drawn attention to differences in patients' and clinicians' perspectives that sometimes give rise to misunderstandings and conflict. Problems may arise due to patients' over-optimistic ideas about the benefits of medical care and doctors' awareness of the limits on what can be achieved (Smith 2001). Smith dubbed this a 'bogus contract', highlighting the need for doctors to tell patients about the limitations and be more open about what they do not know (Figure 8.3).

Exaggerated ideas about the benefits of medical interventions may be due to media influences, commercial pressures or politicians' promises, and they may also be a consequence of paternalistic styles of delivery. This can encourage patients to rely on health professionals to solve their problems, even when this is unrealistic.

Problems may arise due to a failure to tackle the conflicting agendas of clinicians and patients. For example, patients may be anxious about their illness, about whether they will understand the doctor's explanations, or about whether they might be wasting the doctor's time with a trivial problem. Doctors may worry about making an accurate diagnosis, about limiting the duration of the consultation, or about whether their actions would be approved by their peers. These fears remain hidden and are not generally discussed. The consultation process is tightly structured to enable the doctor to retain control, but this can lead to a sense of disempowerment in the patient. Demystifying the process and encouraging greater frankness about what is and is not possible may help, but it must be done sensitively to avoid damaging trust. Trust is built through competence and communication, the aspects of clinical skills that patients value most highly (Calnan and Rowe 2008). 'Competence' includes the ability to display openness, honesty and empathy, as well as technical skills. Many patients are suspicious of clinicians who are not completely frank with them, while others may prefer not to know all the details. Making a judgement about the best approach for a particular individual is one of the most difficult tasks facing those involved in clinical practice.

Learning to work in teams

Nowadays most healthcare is delivered by multidisciplinary teams, yet the curricula for most professional training programmes are unidisciplinary. Health professionals need formal training and practice in teamwork and leadership if they are to provide the type of well-coordinated, integrated care

The bogus contract: the patient's view
- Modern medicine can do remarkable things: it can solve many of my problems
- You, the doctor, can see inside me and know what's wrong
- You know everything it's necessary to know
- You can solve my problems, even my social problems
- So we give you high status and a good salary

The bogus contract: the doctor's view
- Modern medicine has limited powers
- Worse, it's dangerous
- We can't begin to solve all problems, especially social ones
- I don't know everything, but I do know how difficult many things are
- The balance between doing good and harm is very fine
- I'd better keep quiet about all this so as not to disappoint my patients and lose my status

The new contract
Both patients and doctors know:
- Death, sickness, and pain are part of life
- Medicine has limited powers, particularly to solve social problems, and is risky
- Doctors don't know everything: they need decision making and psychological support
- We're in this together
- Patients can't leave problems to doctors
- Doctors should be open about their limitations
- Politicians should refrain from extravagant promises and concentrate on reality.

Source: Reproduced from Smith (2001) with permission from the BMJ Publishing Group Ltd

Figure 8.3 Doctors and patients: redrafting a bogus contract

that most patients want and need. Effective teamworking has been shown to be a key factor in improving health outcomes and reducing errors (Zwarenstein et al. 2009).

A recent WHO report has called for major changes in the way healthcare workers are trained, shifting the emphasis towards interprofessional education and collaborative practice (World Health Organization 2010). Interprofessional education occurs when students from two or more professions learn about, from and with each other. This is said to greatly enhance teamworking because people have a better understanding of each other's roles and professional values and are better able to communicate with each other. While there is some evidence to support this claim, more rigorous research is needed to determine which are the most effective methods for providing interprofessional education (Reeves et al. 2010).

While interprofessional education may be the ideal, some brief interventions have been shown to be effective in improving the way teams work together. For example, surgical checklists that start by asking all staff to introduce themselves to each other have been shown to make a real difference to surgical outcomes (Gawande 2009). Teams work best when they have clear objectives agreed by all team members, effective leadership with flat non-hierarchical structures where everyone is able to express their views, clear protocols and procedures, and effective mechanisms for resolving conflict. Ideally, patients and their families should also be seen as part of the team, with opportunities to participate in team decision-making when appropriate (Canadian Health Services Research Foundation 2006).

The WHO has suggested a series of learning outcomes for interprofessional education (Figure 8.4) (World Health Organization 2010).

---

1 **Teamwork**
   – being able to be both team leader and team member
   – knowing the barriers to teamwork

2 **Roles and responsibilities**
   – understanding one's own roles, responsibilities and expertise, and those of other types of health workers

3 **Communication**
   – expressing one's opinions competently to colleagues
   – listening to team members

4 **Learning and critical reflection**
   – reflecting critically on one's own relationship within a team
   – transferring interprofessional learning to the work setting

5 **Relationship with, and recognizing the needs of, the patient**
   – working collaboratively in the best interests of the patient
   – engaging with patients, their families, carers and communities as partners in care management

6 **Ethical practice**
   – understanding the stereotypical views of other health workers held by self and others
   – acknowledging that each health worker's views are equally valid and important.

Source: Reproduced from the World Health Organization (2010, p. 26) with permission from WHO

Figure 8.4 Learning outcomes for interprofessional education

These skills are practised in workplace settings and can be assessed using structured assessment tools and multisource feedback, including feedback from patients. Workplace-based assessment is considered to be useful because it allows for the evaluation of performance in context for both formative and summative purposes (Miller and Archer 2010). Systematic feedback can improve clinical performance, especially multisource feedback from peers, co-workers and patients. This often involves giving patients brief questionnaires to elicit their views on the performance of individual clinicians. Feedback from patients alone can be useful, but it does not appear to be as effective as multisource feedback from the whole team, including patients (Cheraghi-Sohi and Bower 2008).

Cultural competence

People's health beliefs, attitudes and expectations are influenced by the community in which they live and their cultural background. Culture is shaped by various factors including race, ethnicity, nationality, language, gender, socio-economic status, religion and sexual orientation. Socio-cultural differences can affect people's attitudes to health and illness, their help-seeking behaviour and their response to treatment. They can also influence the way healthcare providers respond to people from different groups, affecting their experiences of receiving healthcare. 'Cultural competence' is the term used to describe the ability of individuals and systems to respond to diverse needs, in particular those of people from minority ethnic groups.

Experience in the USA suggests that cultural competence needs to be tackled at organizational and clinical levels (Betancourt et al. 2002). Healthcare organizations should do all they can to ensure that their services are accessible to people from minority groups; for example, by tackling language barriers, providing interpreters and publishing patient information and signage in minority languages. They should also be alert to discrimination in recruitment, including monitoring the ethnic composition of the workforce. At the clinical level it is recommended that all clinicians should receive cross-cultural training to increase awareness of racial and ethnic health inequalities, teaching them about differences in health beliefs and alerting them to the impact of race, ethnicity and class on clinical decision-making.

Cultural competence is now a core requirement for mental health professionals working with culturally diverse patient groups. In mental healthcare it is particularly important to understand the variety of attitudes and health beliefs of people from culturally diverse populations. Failure to do so can result in diagnostic errors and inappropriate management, in addition to the risk of causing offence and miscommunication. However, as yet there is little information about the effectiveness of cultural competence training in mental health settings. Few studies have been carried out outside North America and very few have evaluated the effects of such training (Bhui et al. 2007).

Most cultural competence training focuses on different perspectives of illness and healing, concepts of race, culture and ethnicity, challenging stereotypes, understanding family and community structures, and overcoming social and language barriers (Mihalic et al. 2010). It is recommended that training includes reflective practice in which trainees can explore their own fears and prejudices and the values and theories that affect their actions (Postgraduate Medical Education and Training Board 2008). It makes sense to focus on the main minority groups that trainees are likely to come across in the local area where they work, but this means they may be less well-equipped to understand the needs of people from other groups. The hope is that they will absorb generic skills for dealing with people from cultures that are different from their own.

Patients as teachers

As we have seen, much education of health professionals takes place in workplace settings where they come into contact with patients. Traditionally patients were involved in teaching only as passive participants; for example, to illustrate symptoms or procedures, but there are clear benefits when patients are given a more active role. Direct contact with patients can help to develop trainees' communication skills, professional attitudes, empathy and clinical reasoning. Active patient participation can be achieved either by using actors as 'simulated patients' or by engaging real patients to talk about their own experiences or to provide formal tuition on particular aspects of the curriculum.

While most patients understand the need for students to receive training in healthcare settings and many are willing to cooperate in teaching sessions, there is a limit to the amount of exposure to inexperienced students that can be inflicted on sick people. To fill the gap it is common to use simulated patients (sometimes called standardized patients). These are people who play the part of real patients in pre-planned scenarios designed to teach diagnostic or communication skills. Professional actors who are 'resting' between jobs, amateur actors with time to spare, and real patients who have recovered from an episode of illness and are willing to talk about their experiences are often employed in this role. Many medical and nursing schools have established banks of simulated patients who they can invite in to help with teaching from time to time. They often get involved in developing the scenarios, drawing on their own personal experience as well as that of other patients and tutors. Simulated patients can also be asked to assess trainees' performance, reporting on whether key competences have been demonstrated within the role play, and in curriculum development.

Scenarios involving simulated patients can be used to give insight into the patient's perspective on their health problem, their health beliefs and the influence of their social circumstances on their ability to look after themselves. Simulated patients can provide constructive feedback, and they may be less reluctant than real patients to express concerns or difficulties about a student's performance. Thompson and colleagues have written about how

In order to realize these benefits it is important to plan carefully for patient involvement. Due attention must be paid to the patient-teacher's emotional well-being and stamina, especially if they have to recount distressing experiences. Students may also find it upsetting to listen to such stories, so their well-being needs to be considered too. Participants must be treated with respect and given full information about what is involved, prior to obtaining their consent (Howe and Anderson 2003). They should be given training, remuneration and appropriate support (Jha et al. 2009). It is considered good practice to invite their feedback on the process, along with that of the students, so as to maintain the focus on high-quality education.

Community-based learning

As an alternative to bringing patients into medical and nursing schools to explain what it feels like to experience an illness and undergo treatment, students have been sent out into the community to follow patient journeys and broaden their experience by meeting and observing patients in general practice and in their own homes (Wass 2009). Learning and practising skills in community settings has been advocated as a good way to teach students and trainees about the realities of people's daily lives and the socio-economic and cultural factors that influence behaviour. Many undergraduate medical programmes have adopted community-based learning or placements, and the need for these seems likely to increase with the current trend towards shifting care out of hospitals and nearer to people's homes.

This practice appears particularly helpful for motivating students in the early years of medical training (Littlewood et al. 2005). Students gain confidence and learn things that cannot be so readily absorbed from reading books or listening to lectures, such as how living conditions affect people's health, how illness impacts on individuals and their families, and the importance of cultural competence and multidisciplinary teamwork. It seems that this early exposure to 'real life' can have a lasting impact on trainees' attitudes to patients and their understanding of communities, greatly enhancing their knowledge of the social determinants of health. If so, perhaps it should be a requirement for all clinicians.

Summary

Health professionals require a broad education in interpersonal skills and the economic, social, environmental and technological factors that impact on people's health, in addition to biological, scientific and technical knowledge. Communication skills can be taught effectively in formal courses, but they must be regularly practised if they are to be maintained. This means learning to overcome obstacles such as inappropriate role models and the pressures of working in stressful environments. Good teamworking is essential for high-quality well-coordinated care and students and trainees need to be able to demonstrate cultural competence. Patients can play a valuable role in the education of health professionals, both as simulated patients acting out a script and as real patients talking about their own experiences. Early exposure to illness in the community can help trainees understand the social determinants of health.

References

Babu, K.S., Law-Min, R., Adlam, T. and Banks, V. (2008) Involving service users and carers in psychiatric education: what do trainees think?, *Psychiatric Bulletin*, 32: 28–31.

Betancourt, J.R., Green, A.R. and Carrillo, J.E. (2002) *Cultural Competence in Health Care: Emerging Frameworks and Practical Approaches*. New York: Commonwealth Fund.

Bhui, K., Warfa, N., Edonya, P., McKenzie, K. and Bhugra, D. (2007) Cultural competence in mental health care: a review of model evaluations, *BMC Health Services Research*, 7: 15.

Bieber, C., Nicolai, J., Hartmann, M., Blumenstiel, K., Ringel, N., Schneider, A., Harter, M., Eich, W. and Loh, A. (2009) Training physicians in shared decision-making – who can be reached and what is achieved?, *Patient Education and Counseling*, 77(1): 48–54.

Bonvicini, K.A., Perlin, M.J., Bylund, C.L., Carroll, G., Rouse, R.A. and Goldstein, M.G. (2009) Impact of communication training on physician expression of empathy in patient encounters, *Patient Education Counseling*, 75(1): 3–10.

Calnan, M. and Rowe, R. (2008) *Trust Matters in Health Care*. Maidenhead: Open University Press.

Campion, P., Foulkes, J., Neighbour, R. and Tate, P. (2002) Patient centredness in the MRCGP video examination: analysis of large cohort, *British Medical Journal*, 325(7366): 691–92.

Canadian Health Services Research Foundation (2006) *Teamwork in Healthcare: Promoting Effective Teamwork in Canada*. Ottawa: Canadian Health Services Research Foundation.

Cheraghi-Sohi, S. and Bower, P. (2008) Can the feedback of patient assessments, brief training, or their combination, improve the interpersonal skills of primary care physicians? A systematic review, *BMC Health Services Research*, 8: 179.

Collins, S., Britten, N., Ruusuvuori, J. and Thompson, A. (2007) *Patient Participation in Health Care Consultations: Qualitative Perspectives*. Maidenhead: Open University Press.

Corke, C.F., Stow, P.J., Green, D.T., Agar, J.W. and Henry, M.J. (2005) How doctors discuss major interventions with high risk patients: an observational study, *British Medical Journal*, 330(7484): 182.

Donaghy, F., Boylan, O. and Loughrey, C. (2010) Using expert patients to deliver teaching in general practice, *British Journal General Practice*, 60(571): 136–39.

Field, K. and Ziebland, S. (2008) 'Beyond the textbook': a preliminary survey of the uses made of the DIPEx website in healthcare education. Available online at www.dipex.org.uk.

Frenk, J., Chen, L., Bhutta, Z.A., Cohen, J., Crisp, N., Evans, T., Fineberg, H., Garcia, P., Ke, Y., Kelley, P., Kistnasamy, B., Meleis, A., Naylor, D., Pablos-Mendez, A., Reddy, S., Scrimshaw, S., Sepulveda, J., Serwadda, D. and Zurayk, H. (2010) Health professionals for a new century: transforming education to strengthen health systems in an interdependent world, *The Lancet*, 376(9756): 1923–58.

Gawande, A. (2009) *The Checklist Manifesto: How to Get Things Right*. London: Profile Books.

General Medical Council (2009a) *Good Medical Practice*. Available online at www.gmc-uk.org. London: GMC.

General Medical Council (2009b) *Tomorrow's Doctors*. Available online at www.gmc-uk.org. London: General Medical Council.

General Medical Council (2010) *Revalidation: The Way Ahead*. London: GMC.

General Pharmaceutical Council (2010) *Standards of Conduct, Ethics and Performance*. Available online at www.pharmacyregulation.org/pdfs/other/gphcstandardsofconductethicsandperflo.pdf.

Gysels, M., Richardson, A. and Higginson, I.J. (2004) Communication training for health professionals who care for patients with cancer: a systematic review of effectiveness, *Supportive Care in Cancer*, 12(10): 692–700.

Hardy, P. (2005) *Patient Voices: An Investigation into Improving the Quality of Healthcare Using Digital Patient Stories*. Cottenham: Pilgrim Projects.

Health Professions Council (2008) *Standards of Conduct, Performance and Ethics*. Available online at www.hpc-uk.org/publications/standards/index.asp?id=38.

Herxheimer, A., McPherson, A., Miller, R., Shepperd, S., Yaphe, J. and Ziebland, S. (2000) Database of patients' experiences (DIPEx): a multi-media approach to sharing experiences and information, *The Lancet*, 355(9214): 1540–43.

Howe, A. and Anderson, J. (2003) Involving patients in medical education, *British Medical Journal*, 327(7410): 326–28.

Jha, V., Quinton, N.D., Bekker, H.L. and Roberts, T.E. (2009) What educators and students really think about using patients as teachers in medical education: a qualitative study, *Medical Education*, 43(5): 449–56.

Kilminster, S., Morris, P., Simpson, E., Thistlethwaite, J. and Eward, B. (2005) Using patients' experiences in medical education: first steps in inter-professional training?, in T. Warne and S. McAndrew (eds), *Using Patient Experience in Nurse Education* (pp. 104–24). Basingstoke: Palgrave Macmillan.

Kleinman, A. (1988) *The Illness Narratives: Suffering, Healing and the Human Condition*. New York: Basic Books.

Kurtz, S., Silverman, J., Benson, J. and Draper, J. (2003) Marrying content and process in clinical method teaching: enhancing the Calgary–Cambridge guides, *Academic Medicine*, 78(8): 802–09.

Lewin, S.A., Skea, Z.C., Entwistle, V., Zwarenstein, M. and Dick, J. (2001) Interventions for providers to promote a patient-centred approach in clinical consultations, *Cochrane Database of Systematic Review*, 4: CD003267.

Littlewood, S., Ypinazar, V., Margolis, S.A., Scherpbier, A., Spencer, J. and Dornan, T. (2005) Early practical experience and the social responsiveness of clinical education: systematic review, *British Medical Journal*, 331(7513): 387–91.

Maguire, P. and Pitceathly, C. (2002) Key communication skills and how to acquire them, *British Medical Journal*, 325(7366): 697–700.

Makoul, G., Zick, A.B., Aakhus, M., Neely, K.J. and Roemer, P.E. (2010) Using an online forum to encourage reflection about difficult conversations in medicine, *Patient Education and Counseling*, 79(1): 83–86.

Mihalic, A.P., Morrow, J.B., Long, R.B. and Dobbie, A.E. (2010) A validated cultural competence curriculum for US pediatric clerkships, *Patient Education and Counseling*, 79(1): 77–82.

Miller, A. and Archer, J. (2010) Impact of workplace based assessment on doctors' education and performance: a systematic review, *British Medical Journal*, 341: c5064.

Nursing and Midwifery Council (2008) *The Code: Standards of Conduct, Performance and Ethics for Nurses and Midwives*. Available online at www.nmc-uk.org.

Nursing and Midwifery Council (2010) *Standards for Pre-registration Nursing Education*. Available online at www.nmc-uk.org.

Owen, C. and Reay, R.E. (2004) Consumers as tutors – legitimate teachers?, *BMC Medical Education*, 4: 14.

Postgraduate Medical Education and Training Board (2008) *Patients Role in Healthcare: The Future Relationship Between Patient and Doctor*. London: PMETB.

Prime Minister's Commission on the Future of Nursing and Midwifery in England. (2010) *Front Line Care: The Future of Nursing and Midwifery in England*. London: Her Majesty's Stationery Office.

Reeves, S., Zwarenstein, M., Goldman, J., Barr, H., Freeth, D., Koppel, I. and Hammick, M. (2010) The effectiveness of interprofessional education: key findings from a new systematic review, *Journal of Interprofessional Care*, 24(3): 230–41.

Royal College of Physicians and Surgeons in Canada (2010) *The CanMEDS Framework*. Canada: Royal College of Physicians and Surgeons in Canada.

Samociuk, G. and McAndrew, S. (2005) A long-term affair, in T. Warne and S. McAndrew (eds), *Using Patient Experience in Nurse Education* (pp. 125–48). Basingstoke: Palgrave Macmillan.

Smith, R. (2001) Why are doctors so unhappy? There are probably many causes, some of them deep, *British Medical Journal*, 322(7294): 1073–74.

Stark, S. and Stronach, I. (2005) Nursing policy paradoxes and educational implications, in T. Warne and S. McAndrew (eds), *Using Patient Experience in Nurse Education* (pp. 63–85). Basingstoke: Palgrave Macmillan.

Stevenson, F.A., Cox, K., Britten, N. and Dundar, Y. (2004) A systematic review of the research on communication between patients and health care professionals about medicines: the consequences for concordance, *Health Expectations*, 7(3): 235–45.

Thompson, B.M., Teal, C.R., Scott, S.M., Manning, S.N., Greenfield, E., Shada, R. and Haidet, P. (2010) Following the clues: teaching medical students to explore patients' contexts, *Patient Education and Counseling*, 80(3): 345–50.

Wass, V. (2009) Extending learning into the community, in Y. Carter and N. Jackson (eds), *Medical Education and Training: From Theory to Delivery* (pp. 79–92). Oxford: Oxford University Press.

World Health Organization (2010) *Framework for Action on Interprofessional Education and Collaborative Practice*. Geneva: WHO Department of Human Resources for Health.

Wykurz, G. and Kelly, D. (2002) Developing the role of patients as teachers: literature review, *British Medical Journal*, 325(7368): 818–21.

Zwarenstein, M., Goldman, J. and Reeves, S. (2009) Interprofessional collaboration: effects of practice-based interventions on professional practice and healthcare outcomes, *Cochrane Database of Systematic Review*, no. 3: CD000072.

Further reading

Carter, Y. and Jackson, N. (eds) (2009) *Medical Education and Training*. Oxford: Oxford University Press.

Collins, S., Britten, N., Ruusuvuori, J. and Thompson, A. (2007) *Patient Participation in Health Care Consultations: Qualitative Perspectives*. Maidenhead: Open University Press.

Kleinman, A. (1988) *The Illness Narratives: Suffering, Healing and the Human Condition*. New York: Basic Books.

Warne, T. and McAndrew, S. (2005) *Using Patient Experience in Nurse Education*. Basingstoke: Palgrave Macmillan.

9 | **Shaping services**

Overview

In this chapter we look at what can be achieved when groups of people work together to improve health and care. After a brief discussion of why collective engagement is considered important, we look at the role and impact of patient organizations, both voluntary and statutory, and at community groups. This is followed by a description of how healthcare commissioners have engaged with local groups to determine health needs, to promote health, to improve service design and to decide on spending priorities. Finally, we look at lay involvement in the governance of healthcare bodies and their accountability to local people.

Social capital, co-production and participatory democracy

Why is it important to encourage citizen involvement in shaping health policy and practice? Those who argue that fostering collective engagement is an important role for governments, health authorities and healthcare commissioners often refer to benefits that can accrue from building community cohesion or social capital. Social capital is a way of describing the norms, networks and interactions (sense of belonging) that facilitate collective action (Putnam 2000). Many commentators consider it essential for economic development and for fostering inclusion and social cohesion, as well as being the key to tackling health inequalities (Health Development Agency 2004b). Advocates argue that groups and communities are best placed to articulate their health needs and they should therefore be given the opportunity to shape health service provision.

There is also a belief that co-production (delivering services in an equal and reciprocal relationship between professionals, patients, their families and communities) will lead to more responsive services and better health outcomes (Boyle et al. 2010; National Institute for Clinical Excellence 2008). Co-production can operate both at the collective level with citizens actively participating in key decisions; for example, about resource allocation priorities or resolving ethical dilemmas and at the individual level between patients and clinicians (Tudor Hart 2010). The output or product of effective co-production is health gain, including gains in life expectancy, relief of painful and debilitating symptoms, improved quality of life, emotional health and sense of well-being. Co-production recognizes that citizens and communities have assets or capabilities that can be mobilized. The 'community asset' model aims to build on these resources, focusing on what people can do instead of seeking to make up for what they cannot do (Improvement and Development Agency 2010).

Albert Weale has outlined six reasons for fostering citizen involvement or participatory democracy in healthcare (Weale 2006):

1 Planning services from the user point of view – this should go beyond the specific group of people who use the service to take account of competing priorities.
2 Improving the technical quality of decisions – members of the public can contribute additional perspectives and alternative ways of appraising policy options to complement those of the professionals most closely involved.
3 Consulting co-producers – because citizens make important contributions to public health, they have a right to be consulted and listened to.
4 Rectifying an imbalance of policy influence – since the NHS is virtually a monopoly provider, producer interests are very powerful. Encouraging citizen participation is necessary to redress the power imbalance.
5 Avoiding unnecessary confrontation and creating the conditions for consensus – to enhance the legitimacy of policy choices it is important to ensure a fair and open decision-making process.
6 Identifying competing perspectives on issues, particularly in respect of their moral dimensions – health policy-makers often face decisions which raise complex ethical issues; for example, abortion or stem cell therapy. In these cases it is particularly important to test assumptions with a widely representative range of citizens.

The arguments are appealing, but implementing collective engagement and measuring its effects is not straightforward. On the face of it people appear to welcome the opportunity to get engaged, at least hypothetically. The vast majority of people – 90 per cent in one survey – felt local people should have a say in how the NHS is run (Developing Patient Partnerships 2006). But in another survey only 22 per cent said they wanted to be actively involved themselves in planning or delivering services (Audit Commission 2003). And the proportion who actually do get involved in practice when invited to do so often shrinks to a tiny, unrepresentative minority (Skidmore et al. 2006). Community participation tends to be dominated by a small group of people willing to get involved in a range of community activities. Any social capital created by opening up governance to lay involvement tends to be concentrated in the hands of this minority. While they undoubtedly play a valuable role, there is no guarantee that the wider community feels the benefit of this social capital. The efforts of this group need to be supplemented by a wider range of engagement methods. These may involve statutory organizations reaching out to people and devolving some of their power to local community groups.

Engaging with local communities is more difficult than it may at first appear, but by no means impossible. Later in this chapter we look at some examples of how this has been tackled and at techniques that can be used to encourage participation.

Early patient groups

Since the nineteenth century people have formed groups to fund-raise and campaign for improvements in the quality of healthcare. Initially many of those arguing for reform were health professionals. Florence Nightingale used all the techniques of a modern-day community activist – publicizing suffering, advocacy, data-gathering, networking, fund-raising and political lobbying – to enlist support for her campaigns to improve healthcare for the poor in London and for soldiers fighting in Crimea (Bostridge 2008). Other prominent individuals have played a key role in mobilizing public opinion. Twentieth-century writers drew attention to the shortcomings of healthcare, including George Bernard Shaw (Shaw 1906), Erving Goffman (Goffman 1961), Ivan Illich (Illich 1974) and Thomas McKeown (McKeown 1976). Their critiques encouraged others to challenge traditional ways of organizing care.

Roy Porter traced the origins of today's patient groups to 'the 1960s populist counter-culture backlash against scientific and technological arrogance' (Porter 2003: 167–68). People began to question the overweening power of the medical establishment and groups were established to campaign for patients' rights. Some of these groups were highly influential and long-lived. For example, Mother Care for Children in Hospital, founded in 1961 by a group of parents, was later renamed the National Association for the Welfare of Children in Hospital and is still going strong under its new name, Action for Sick Children. The charity was established in response to concern about the then common practice of separating children from their parents during long hospital stays. Despite the publication of a government report arguing that the practice should cease, almost no change ensued until the organization organized a highly effective campaign that mobilized wider public opinion. The battle to lift restrictions on parents' visiting hours was eventually won in 1986, since when the group has gone on to campaign for further improvements in the care of sick children.

Other groups had their origins in the women's movement, stimulated by the writings of American feminists who were highly critical of the medical profession's domination of healthcare and promoted the idea of mutual self-help and demystification of medical knowledge (Ehrenreich and English 2010). In 1973 a groundbreaking book was published in the USA entitled *Our Bodies, Ourselves* that confronted women's ignorance of their bodies by providing them with educational material and guidance on self-care (Boston Women's Health Book Collective 1998). The book was updated and reprinted numerous times, translated into many different languages and distributed worldwide, informing and educating hundreds of thousands of women over more than a quarter of a century.

Growth of patient organizations

The 1980s saw rapid growth in the number of patient organizations and this expansion continues to the present day. A search of the website of the Charity Commission for England and Wales using the keyword 'patients' yields the names of more than a thousand charitable organizations concerned with improving healthcare for patients. Not all of these are patient-led or grass-roots groups – some were established by health professionals and others are charitable foundations attached to hospitals – but the growth in numbers of voluntary sector groups is a reflection of the huge public interest in health and healthcare.

The majority of patient organizations focus their efforts on a single condition or linked group of conditions, such as cancer, heart disease, diabetes or mental health. Others represent the interests of specific sub-groups of the population; for example, children, older people or minority ethnic groups. A smaller proportion are generic, covering all healthcare issues. These include statutory organizations established by government to represent patients' interests and patient participation groups in general practice. There are also a few alliances or umbrella groups that represent the collective interests of their member organizations.

Most voluntary patient organizations are membership bodies with boards of trustees and formal articles of association, prerequisites for charitable registration. They fund themselves by levying subscription fees, as well as seeking sponsorships, grants and donations. Most engage in a range of activities, including awareness-raising and campaigning, provision of information and advice, supporting research and providing goods and services. They range in size, from small local groups with limited ambitions and reach, to large professionally run organizations, involving both health professionals and laypeople among their managers, advisers and trustees. The largest have networks of local groups and turnovers running into millions of pounds.

Patient participation groups in general practice (PPGs) have a fairly long history, dating back to the early 1970s. The National Association for Patient Partnership was founded in 1978 and is still going strong, with nearly 500 affiliated groups. Most PPGs were initiated by GPs and they engage in a variety of activities including the provision of services, for example, transport and prescription collection schemes, visiting and befriending, running crèches and fund-raising; providing feedback about practice organization (including suggestion boxes, surveys and open meetings), and health promotion or community development (including lectures, discussion groups, self-help groups and campaigning on local issues). Some PPGs are now getting involved in helping GP commissioners to determine the needs and views of local communities. However, it is hard for these groups to persuade large numbers of patients to get involved and those that do are often not representative of the practice population.

Influencing policy

In recent years the role of patient organizations has attracted the attention of political scientists and sociologists who saw them as a potentially significant influence on public policy. Bruce Wood carried out a cross-national comparison of disease-related patient groups in Britain and the USA (Wood 2000). In both countries he found a large assortment of groups engaged in providing services and voicing the concerns of their members. Many acted as pressure groups, increasing public awareness of the special needs of their members and influencing the distribution of resources for healthcare and medical research. However, their efforts were often fragmented and unco-ordinated, with many groups covering overlapping territory and competing for funding and support. This fragmentation was held to be responsible for their relatively weak influence on health policy, as compared to that of other stakeholders, including doctors, managers and industry.

A slightly later British study documented signs of more collaborative relationships, with the emergence of alliances between patient organizations (Baggott et al. 2005). Most of the groups studied were involved in some kind of network with like-minded organizations, both informal alliances and organized umbrella groups. The authors found evidence of a broader national and even international patient 'movement', resulting from a perception of shared interests and an awareness that greater strength lay in collaboration. Collaboration was not without its difficulties, however. Many organizations competed for funding from the same or similar sources and their success depended on having a high media profile and brand awareness. This tended to inhibit the desire to combine forces.

Values and priorities sometimes collided too. For example, some organizations were suspicious of the willingness of rival groups to collaborate closely with health professionals. Others were nervous of the political stance of their rivals, and there were disagreements about the wisdom of accepting donations from pharmaceutical or biotechnology companies. The issue of funding has been the subject of wide debate, attracting criticism of some patient organizations for failing to be transparent about their funding sources. Some people argued that accepting money from commercial sources exposed the groups to a conflict of interest that they could not control and risked co-option by commercial interests, while others felt there was nothing unacceptable in the practice (Kent 2007; Mintzes 2007).

While the combined resources of patient organizations are substantial, few can hope to counter the much greater resources available to industry and professional groups. Developing strategic alliances with other groups and stakeholders makes sense, as long as there are safeguards in place to maintain organizational integrity when interests diverge.

Community Health Councils

While voluntary patient organizations have made important contributions to public policy, it is clear that they represent sectional interests only and cannot be expected to speak for the whole population. In an attempt to redress the balance, successive governments have provided financial support to establish statutory patient organizations. Groups set up with public funds have been established in various countries, including Australia, Germany, the Netherlands and the UK. The history of statutory patient groups in England illustrates the problematic nature of sustaining population-based initiatives in the face of government ambivalence about transferring real power to citizens.

Community Health Councils (CHCs) were established in 1974 to represent patients' interests at local level. There were 182 CHCs in England, each of which had 18 members appointed by local health authorities, local councils and the voluntary sector. Wholly funded by the Department of Health – albeit not very generously – they were independent of local healthcare providers. They had a statutory right to be consulted about major service redevelopments and a legal duty to monitor services by inspecting premises, reviewing performance and assisting complainants. Beyond this their role was not clearly defined. It was never entirely clear whether CHCs were supposed to act as consumer watchdogs representing the interests of local patients, or as a form of participatory democracy designed to increase citizen representation in policy-making (Klein 2001). Many tried to balance both these roles by engaging in diverse activities, including helping people make formal complaints about their care, preparing detailed comments on local plans, and working with local agencies to promote public health.

During their 30-year existence some CHCs succeeded in making considerable impact at local level, but others were less successful (Hogg 2009). Lacking formal procedures for election to their boards, they were largely dependent on the energy and commitment of unpaid volunteers, often those with a specific vested interest, and a very small number of paid staff. To some extent their role was undermined by successive waves of policy innovation in which, for example, health authorities were given lead responsibility for public consultation and alternative systems for dealing with complaints were established.

New statutory groups

Eventually, in 2003 CHCs were abolished by the government and replaced by 572 Patient and Public Involvement Forums, each linked to a healthcare provider organization, and by Health Overview and Scrutiny Committees in each local authority. The reorganization was ill-fated from the start. The cumbersome arrangements for establishing the new groups ran into problems almost immediately and the body that was supposed to coordinate their efforts and provide support, the Commission for Patient and Public Involvement in Health (CPPIH), faced difficulties with funding, management and political support. CHC activists opposed the changes and forums were slow to get established, with many finding it difficult to recruit and retain members. The whole structure was viewed as unsatisfactory by its critics, mainly because the forums had weaker powers and less independence than the CHCs they replaced. The abolition of CPPIH was announced by the government in July 2004, a mere 20 months after it began work. A couple of years later in July 2006 the demise of the forums was also signalled. They were to be replaced by yet another raft of statutory patient/user groups known as Local Involvement Networks (LINks).

LINks were not attached to specific provider organizations. Instead each of the 150 local authorities was required to make arrangements to establish a LINk which was expected to represent the interests of users of both health and social care services in a their local area. The government hoped they would focus their attention on health and social care commissioning rather than service provision. However, they had almost no time to show what they could achieve before further change was introduced. The coalition government that came to power in May 2010 announced that it intended 'to strengthen the collective voice of patients' by introducing a new national body, to be known as HealthWatch England. This was to be established within the Care Quality Commission, the body responsible for regulating quality in health and social care provider organizations, and HealthWatch was to be the consumer watchdog (Secretary of State for Health 2010). LINks were to be transformed into local HealthWatch groups, reporting to and coordinated by the national body.

Reviewing the messy history of the statutory groups, Christine Hogg argued that the effect of the various reorganizations was to reduce local public influence on health policy-making (Hogg 2009). If the government's true aim was to foster participatory democracy, they had gone about it in an odd way. The statutory groups were never given sufficient resources to do a really effective job and there was continuing confusion about their powers and responsibilities. The government appeared more interested in fostering consumerism than in strengthening civil society, and tinkering with the structures had done little to effect a transfer of power to citizens.

Community groups

The term 'community' can mean a number of things. According to the *Shorter Oxford English Dictionary* it can refer to 'an organized political, municipal, or social body'; 'a body of people living in the same locality'; 'a body of people having religion, profession etc. in common'; 'a sense of common identity' (Oxford University Press 2007). It encompasses not just geographical communities, but also people sharing a common identity by reason of their faith, ethnic origin, occupation, organizational affiliation, health status, disability, and so on. There is undoubtedly some overlap between community groups and patient organizations. Many community groups are interested in health issues, but they tend to be looser or less formal in structure and are often focused on small geographical areas.

Most communities have a plethora of groups, including residents' associations, youth groups, sports groups, pensioners' groups, and local groups affiliated to national organizations. Some community groups come into being as a result of external stimulus from a local authority or neighbourhood worker with a brief to consult or engage local people. There are divided views on the appropriate focus for community engagement in health. Some people advocate working with groups of disadvantaged people in specific locations, such as a housing estate, encouraging them to address any or all of their concerns which may include economic development, employment, housing, education and training, and so on. This builds on a long tradition of community development, espousing a holistic or social model to empower communities. Community members are encouraged to set the agenda to tackle the issues that they deem most important. Of course, these issues may not necessarily involve health or healthcare directly, but helping people to take action to improve their lives may strengthen community cohesion or social capital which may in turn have an impact on people's health.

Involvement in commissioning

Healthcare commissioners (the bodies responsible for planning health services for a local population and allocating resources) tend to see their responsibilities to engage with their local communities somewhat differently from the community development specialists. Their concern is to respond to the healthcare needs of people living in their catchment area and to improve local services by learning from the experience of service users. So they usually prefer to cast a wider geographical net that encompasses the whole of the local health economy. Their main contacts tend to be with representatives of organized community groups and they often control the agenda to ensure a focus on health and healthcare.

Commentators on community engagement are fond of referring to a model of participation known as Arnstein's ladder. Developed by Sherry Arnstein, a public policy analyst who studied citizen involvement in urban planning in the USA, this conceptual framework categorized levels of involvement according to the amount of power that is transferred to citizens (Arnstein 1969). The levels range from lay membership of committees, deemed tokenism or manipulation by Arnstein, through to community control of facilities and services. This hierarchical approach may have its uses for understanding involvement in urban development, but it has proved less useful for categorizing the range of approaches used nowadays to engage communities in health policy. An updated version of the ladder, developed by Contra Costa Health Services in California, is more helpful as a way of describing the different types and roles of community engagement that can help to shape healthcare (Morgan and Lifshay 2006) (Figure 9.1).

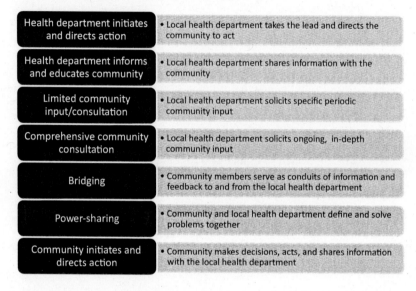

Source: Adapted from Morgan and Lifsay (2006) with permission from Contra Costa Health Services

Figure 9.1 Ladder of community participation

When thinking about community engagement in healthcare commissioning, for example, a comprehensive community consultation may be necessary if a major reorganization is planned, but often input from a number of community leaders will suffice, acting in a bridging role to provide information and feedback to their local groups. Contra Costa Health Services caution against seeing the Ladder of Community Participation as a hierarchy of desirability, where the first rung of the ladder is seen as the least desirable. Instead it is conceived as a planning tool to help organizations decide where to start the process of community engagement and where they hope to get to. Goals and starting points will differ according to the context and capacity in the local community.

Another way of looking at community participation in commissioning is to see it as a continuous cycle of activities. The Engagement Cycle is a way of classifying the various ways in which local people can be involved, including helping to identify local needs and aspirations, developing strategic priorities and plans, designing and improving services, procuring and contracting services, to monitoring and managing performance (InHealth Associates 2009).

Some primary care trusts in England have managed to involve laypeople in each of these activities.

Accountability

The NHS Constitution makes several important pledges to patients and members of the public in England, including the following:

> You have the right to be involved, directly or through representatives, in the planning of healthcare services, the development and consideration of proposals for changes in the way those services are provided, and in decisions to be made affecting the operation of those services.
>
> The NHS also commits to provide you with the information you need to influence and scrutinise the planning and delivery of NHS services (pledge); and to work in partnership with you, your family, carers and representatives (pledge).
>
> (Department of Health 2009: 7)

These rights and pledges place a duty on NHS organizations to involve laypeople in governance, to ensure transparency of decision-making, and to be accountable to citizens.

Accountability is distinct from public involvement. It requires organizations to provide information and give explanations for their decisions. Local representatives must be able to interrogate those responsible and require answers, with sanctions that can be invoked if they are dissatisfied with their conduct (Local Government Association Health Commission 2008). In other words, accountability requires a formal process, whereas public consultation or engagement relies on informal mechanisms. However, one of the important aspects for which public organizations should be held to account is the extent to which they have engaged with members of their local communities.

There are three main domains of public services for which good governance and public accountability is felt to be essential:

1 financial accountability – value for money
2 accountability for performance – quality of services
3 political and democratic accountability – responsiveness to service users
   (Centre for Public Scrutiny 2007).

The traditional model of public accountability was upwards to Parliament or Whitehall, but nowadays this is felt to be insufficient. Representative democracy – allowing the electorate the chance to express their views at the ballot box once every four or five years – is not enough to ensure that public services respond adequately to people's needs and desires. The highly centralised system of accountability in the NHS has been described as 'strong nationally and weak, or non-existent, at local level' (Local Government Association Health Commission 2008: 2).

Recognition that the centrally funded and directed NHS suffered from a democratic deficit led to a search for new forms of local accountability. The renewed emphasis on community engagement is part of this shift in thinking. Mechanisms such as local strategic partnerships, coupled with a legal duty to involve local people, were introduced in an attempt to ensure that services retained public support and responded to local perceptions of needs and priorities (Department of Health 2008).

Governance

Governance has been defined as:

> The system by which an organisation is directed and controlled, at its most senior levels, in order to achieve its objectives and meet the necessary standards of accountability and probity.
>
> (Cadbury Report 1992: 2.5).

Governance in the public sector in general, and the NHS in particular, has made great strides in England in recent years, especially in the involvement of laypeople. Legislation opened up various opportunities for members of the public to get involved in the governance of healthcare organizations. All NHS trusts (healthcare provider organizations) now have boards made up of executive and non-executive directors, with non-executives, one of whom is the board chair, comprising a majority. Boards have collective responsibility for formulating strategy, holding the organization to account and shaping its culture. Most non-executive directors are laypeople with specific skills required by the board. The board is expected to adhere to the seven principles of public life (National Leadership Centre Board Development 2010):

1 selflessness
2 integrity
3 objectivity
4 accountability
5 openness
6 honesty
7 leadership.

Boards of NHS trusts are not elected and their meetings are not always open to the public. They are directly accountable to strategic health authorities and the Department of Health, but there are few formal mechanisms to underscore their accountability to local people. This is changing, however, with the establishment of foundation trusts. These are public interest companies owned by their members, made up of local people and staff who choose to sign up. Members elect boards of governors to represent their interests and hold the board of directors to account. The government's intention in introducing this new form of ownership was to make the foundation trusts accountable to their local communities instead of upwards to the Secretary of State for Health. However, the government has consistently resisted calls to hand over control of health services to democratically elected local authorities, as happens in several other European countries (Blackman et al. 2008).

Engagement methods

With the introduction of a purchaser–provider split in the NHS, those responsible for commissioning healthcare were expected to make careful assessments of local needs, ensuring that local services were responsive to local people. They were required to work with local authorities, voluntary organizations and other agencies in strategic partnerships to develop joint strategic needs assessments to guide health improvements (Department of Health 2007). The goal was to ensure that the NHS was locally accountable and shaped by the people who used it. Doing the job properly involved keeping in touch with the views of all local residents, not just the small minority who turned out for public meetings or volunteered to sit on committees. In particular commissioners were enjoined to reach out to minority or disadvantaged groups whose views may be ignored unless special efforts are made to listen to them. This was no easy task. Many primary care trusts and practice-based commissioners lacked the skills, experience and confidence to do this effectively (Picker Institute Europe 2009).

Sometimes described pejoratively as 'the usual suspects', the select group of people who respond to invitations to join planning groups or volunteer to sit on policy committees undoubtedly have an important contribution to make. Often these people are already involved in other organizations, such as patient groups. They may be well placed to articulate the perspective of their organization and its members, but they cannot be expected to represent the diversity of views among the much larger population of service users. Other ways must be devised to ensure that a more representative selection of the views of the local community, including those likely to be affected by the issue under question, is heard and taken into account.

A wide range of methods has been advocated for securing community engagement – from informing and consulting through to full community control. In general we lack a critical literature and sufficiently rigorous evaluations to provide definitive guidance on which techniques are most appropriate for which purpose (Smith et al. 2009). Nevertheless, there is much to be learnt from the experience of those who have tried it and several specialist organizations have produced helpful guidance.

Involve, an organization set up to promote community engagement, lists various tools and techniques that have been developed to assist in public participation (Involve and togetherwecan 2005). Some of the most commonly used methods are listed in Figure 9.2.

Most successful efforts to engage with local people involve a plurality of methods carefully selected to fit the task at hand (Involve 2010). Which to

Techniques for use with large groups	Techniques for use with smaller groups	Online techniques for use with those who have Internet access
Twenty first-century town meeting	Appreciative inquiry	Blogs
Area forums	Citizen advisory groups	ePanels
Citizen's summit	Citizen's panels	Online consultations
Community development	Citizen's jury	Online forum
Consensus conference	Café consultation	Twitter
Deliberative mapping	Customer journey mapping	Webcasting
Deliberative polling	Deliberative workshops	Web chat
Fun days/festivals	Delphi survey	Wiki
Future search	Focus groups	
Open space events	Mystery shopping	
Opinion polls	Participatory appraisal	
Surveys	Participatory strategic planning	
	Planning for real	
	User panels	

Source: Involve (2010), www.peopleandparticipation.net

Figure 9.2 Participatory methods

choose depends on what you are trying to achieve and the type of participants you want to attract, as well as practical issues such as the resources
and time available. As an alternative to the traditional public meeting in a
draughty village hall, many healthcare organizations have organized fun-
days and other informal events that attract people wanting an enjoyable
day out, as well as giving them an opportunity to have their say on key local issues. Consensus conferences are useful for examining a topic in depth,
such as a new scientific or technological development, and they usually offer laypeople opportunities to question expert witnesses. Deliberative techniques such as citizen's juries or polls aim to engage people in thinking
through controversial policy options, examining them in a similar fashion
to the way juries in criminal courts sift through the evidence. Electronic panels are a much cheaper way to obtain people's views, but of course can only
be used by those with Internet access.

Each of these methods can be used effectively to encourage engagement
with health topics, but the key to success is knowing why you want people
to participate. As the experts at Involve put it:

The most important factor for practitioners is to be clear about why they are doing it in a particular instance, to communicate that to all participants and to agree it with them. Lack of clarity is one of the biggest causes of participation failure.

(Involve and togetherwecan 2005: 21)

In the following sections we look at some examples of what different health-care organizations have done to engage with their local populations.

Determining local needs and aspirations

Health needs assessment has been defined as 'a systematic method for re-viewing the health issues facing a population, leading to agreed priorities and resource allocation that will improve health and reduce inequalities (National Institute for Clinical Excellence 2009: 6).' It is the first step in a commissioning cycle that includes assessing needs, reviewing services and identifying gaps, analysing health risks, deciding on priorities, determining strategic options, implementing contracts, developing providers and man-aging provider performance.

There is nothing new about needs assessment – public health specialists have been producing statistical analyses and epidemiological profiles for many years and these have informed commissioning plans and local health im-provement strategies. Nowadays, however, there is an expectation that the statistical analyses and options appraisals will be accompanied by, and take account of, extensive consultation with local people. Commissioners are expected to ensure that their local strategies are built on an in-depth under-standing of the needs and aspirations of all sections of the local community. This may require the development of different methods of investigation, including those led and carried out by members of the community them-selves. The best local consultations involve a variety of methods to ensure that the diversity of perspectives is understood and all sections of the com-munity have an opportunity to give their views. Feeding back the results to participants once the consultation process is complete is considered equally important.

In the process of developing its strategy for primary and community care, Liverpool Primary Care Trust (PCT) organized a three-stage community con-sultation, entitled the Big Health Debate (Liverpool Primary Care Trust 2007). As well as organizing various surveys, PCT staff visited more than 40 commu-nity groups and then organized a one-day deliberative event for 150 partic-ipants. This event helped to gauge reactions to various options for change. Special efforts were made to seek out the views of minority groups, including people from the Chinese, Sikh, Somali and Yemeni communities, home-less men, Irish travellers, people with sensory disabilities and mental health service users. A further survey of more than 600 regular users of primary care services provided additional information on local people's responses to reorganization plans. A series of workshops was organized to determine the views of health professionals. The conclusions of the consultation, which had involved a total of 11 000 people, were incorporated into the PCT's health strategy and a final public meeting was organized to feed back the results to participants. The reward for these efforts was increased public acceptance of the need for change and an enhanced sense of local ownership of the reorganization plans.

Some projects have gone beyond traditional methods of professionally led consultation to involve local community members in leading the process. For example, a social care charity, Turning Point, developed a vision for integrating health, housing and social care in the most deprived communities with the community playing a central role in the design and delivery of those services (Turning Point 2010). Turning Point's Connected Care programme promoted community audits in which local people were recruited to find out what other local people thought about local services. The idea was to support local people in developing their own needs assessment or community profile. The first pilot took place in one ward in Hartlepool in the north-west of England. The ward was ranked as one of the most deprived nationally, with most residents living in social housing, but it had a well-developed community and voluntary sector with strong residents' associations. Auditors were recruited from these groups and trained to carry out the audit. The audit involved an initial survey, followed by one-to-one interviews, focus groups and a 'Have your say' event. In total 251 people participated in the process. An evaluation of the project pointed to a number of important learning points, including strategies for overcoming initial difficulties in recruiting community members to join the project, the need for a flexible approach to payment for volunteers, and the need for professional staff to work alongside the community auditors to ensure the final report was written and delivered within the agreed timescale (Callaghan and Duggan 2008). Having identified local needs, Turning Point went on to explore new ways of meeting them, including the appointment of citizen adviser schemes to help people interact successfully with public services (Kramer 2010).

Deciding on spending priorities

As healthcare commissioners, Primary Care Trusts (PCTs) have a statutory duty to promote the health of their local communities, but they must do this without exceeding their annual financial allocation. These legal requirements mean that from time to time difficult choices have to be made. Taking decisions about the quality, availability, design and funding of local services can lead healthcare commissioners into controversial waters, especially when this involves denying services to particular groups or individuals. Commissioning bodies should develop coherent principles to guide their decision-making. These will have most legitimacy when they are developed with the active involvement of local people and the rationale for decisions is communicated effectively.

Daniels and Sabin have developed a set of principles to guide those responsible for determining priorities for resource allocation in healthcare, entitled 'accountability for reasonableness' (Daniels and Sabin 1998). They suggest that decision-makers should pay attention to four conditions or principles to maximize the chance of achieving local buy-in:

1 **Publicity**: The public has access to both the decisions and the rationales for priority-setting.
2 **Relevance**: The rationales should be acceptable by 'fair-minded' people as a way of providing value for money while meeting health needs for a defined population under resource constraints.
3 **Appeals**: There must be ways to challenge decisions and resolve disputes, and these must offer an opportunity to revise decisions; for example, in the light of new evidence.
4 **Enforcement**: Action to ensure the first three conditions are met through either voluntary or mandatory regulation.

These principles are widely accepted, at least in theory, but healthcare commissioners in England have often failed to follow the guidance (Robert 2003). In many cases the basis for their decisions is not well communicated and appeals procedures are not well established. However, Oxfordshire PCT, along with others in the Thames Valley, has tackled the issue by establishing a priorities forum. This has developed an explicit ethical framework to guide decisions about which 'exceptional' treatments should be funded. This gives priority to evidence of clinical and cost-effectiveness, equity, healthcare need and capacity to benefit, and patient choice. The framework was developed in consultation with local people and is published on the PCT's website. This does not eliminate public protests when individuals are denied treatment, but it does enable the PCT to demonstrate that its procedures conform to the requirements of accountability for reasonableness.

Various techniques can be used to secure active engagement of local people in priority-setting, including citizen's panels, citizen's juries, deliberative forums and others. In addition a number of practical exercises have been devised to elicit people's values and preferences when faced with rationing decisions or policy options. These techniques are designed for use when there is lack of consensus on the best way forward and a formal evaluation of people's views is felt to be necessary. They include voting, ranking, rating and scaling and techniques such as budget pie, paired comparisons, standard gamble and willingness to pay (Mullen 1999). Choice of technique depends on the topic and the participants. The exercise must be easy to understand and participants must be willing to 'play the game'. They can be useful when there are important trade-offs to be made between benefits and risks, or when a policy question touches on ethical issues about which people may have strong and divergent views.

One such example tackled the issue of flour fortification. The question of whether flour should be fortified with folic acid to reduce the incidence of neural tube defects in newborn babies is an example of a difficult trade-off. Fortification of flour could reduce the incidence of spina bifida and anencephaly, which affect about 180 babies in the UK each year, but it might lead to a delay in diagnosis for some elderly people with vitamin B_{12} deficiency because the higher levels of folic acid can mask the disease, which causes some loss of sensation in arms and legs. A consultation exercise to find out what people felt about this issue and the intensity of their feelings used a household survey that included a willingness-to-pay exercise, a policy vote and open-ended questions asking respondents to give the reasons for their decisions (Dixon and Shackley 2003). People were asked whether they would be willing to contribute anything extra in taxation to allow fortification to go ahead and if so, how much. The willingness-to-pay exercise showed that while a majority were in favour of fortification, only half of these were willing to pay for it in increased taxes. The use of techniques such as willingness to pay gave an indication of the strength of their feelings.

Public engagement with policy dilemmas can lead to improved knowledge and understanding among those directly involved and the results of their deliberations can be influential, but they are often costly and time-consuming to organize (Abelson et al. 2003). Whether the benefits justify the costs requires further research, but their usefulness depends in large part on what policy-making bodies do with the resulting recommendations.

Service development

Many community engagement projects have service improvement and re-design as a central focus. Since almost everyone uses the health service from time to time, most discussions about health needs inevitably come round to people's concerns about the quality of local service provision and gaps in the availability of particular services. Engaging local people and service users in quality improvement efforts requires considerable effort on the part of NHS organizations. Most members of the public do not know how they could get involved in shaping local services if they wanted to and in general most people do not come forward to talk about their experiences or give their views without a great deal of encouragement. In a 2005 survey, only 10 per cent of respondents said they knew how to get involved in making decisions about local health services (e.g. by attending meetings or joining a local patients group) (Healthcare Commission 2005).

Instead of waiting for local residents to initiate ideas for new services, in a few places social entrepreneurs have seized the initiative and invited local people to join them. Bromley by Bow Centre in the London Borough of Tower Hamlets was established in 1984 when Revd Andrew Mawson became minister of the local United Reformed Church. He found a dwindling, elderly congregation and recognized that if the church was to survive it had to adopt a different approach. He persuaded his congregation to open up the building to the local community. Local artists became involved and agreed to teach their skills in return for rent-free workshops, the church started a nursery and the building was used for a variety of events, including Eid and May Day celebrations, Chinese New Year and harvest suppers. As it grew beyond the church, Bromley by Bow Centre developed as a secular organization in its own right, expanding to include a health centre staffed by general practitioners and nurses. By 2010 it had a turnover of more than £3 million a year and employed more than 100 staff. It was the third largest provider of adult education in the borough and provided services to more than 2,000 people each week, including families, young people, vulnerable adults and elders. Bromley by Bow Centre is an example of bottom-up service development that is rooted in an understanding of the needs of the local community. The project leadership was able to act opportunistically to fill gaps in state provision, working in partnership with local statutory and voluntary organizations to regenerate the area where it is located.

Promoting health and reducing inequalities

Many organizations with a specific focus on community engagement list improving health and reducing inequalities among their goals. Some of the most successful projects have emerged from communities that have a clear identity and focused goals rooted in an understanding of specific health needs; for example, those involving minority ethnic groups (Kai and Hedges 1999).

The impact of involving patient organizations or community groups on health outcomes is hard to gauge precisely. There are some impressive examples of successful community-based projects; for example, the North Karelia project in Finland which aimed to prevent cardiovascular disease among a population that suffered the highest rate of mortality from this cause in the world (Puska 2008). The programme involved community leaders, voluntary organizations, the food industry, sports and agricultural groups and healthcare staff working together to mobilize health promotion efforts in villages, schools, workplaces and local media. Early results were encouraging and after five years the programme was expanded to cover the rest of Finland. Cardiovascular mortality rates for men aged 35–64 fell by 79 per cent between 1969 to 2006 and there were significant improvements in the adoption of healthier eating habits.

The multi-pronged nature of the North Karelia project illustrates why it is difficult to determine the effect of community engagement with any precision. Isolating its impact from those of other factors, including wider economic and social influences on health behaviours, is difficult. Few studies of the effectiveness of health promotion initiatives have compared community-based approaches against other methods, such as legislation, mass communication or direct provision of lifestyle advice. There is evidence of a persistent gap between rich and poor in relation to a plethora of health indicators (Marmot 2009). Carefully targeted health promotion programmes and social marketing can reduce health risks in certain groups, but very little is known about the extent to which they reduce health inequalities *between* groups.

One of the most extensive and ambitious attempts to develop community engagement initiatives across the UK was the Health Action Zone (HAZ) programme launched by the government in 1997. Twenty-six HAZs were set up with the intention of monitoring their progress over seven years. They were meant not only to improve health outcomes and reduce health inequalities, but also to act as trailblazers for new ways of working at a local level (Health Development Agency 2004a). However, central government funding for the programme ceased before the end of the allotted time period and an evaluation found that it had produced mixed results. Many of the HAZs succeeded in focusing local attention on health improvement and inequalities, but there was disappointingly little evidence of an impact on reducing the health gap between social groups.

A more recent initiative, the Healthy Communities Programme, suggested that focusing on carefully defined and precise goals may produce better results. Members of local communities were recruited to join a collaborative project designed to improve health and wellbeing (Slater et al. 2008). They attended learning workshops during which they learnt about change principles and how to apply these in a local context. An early focus of the programme was on reducing falls in older people. In three sites covering a population of 150 000 they documented a 32 per cent reduction in falls as a result of community initiatives (730 fewer falls over two years). The project team estimated that this initiative had reduced hospital costs by £1.2 million, ambulance costs by £120 000 and costs of residential social care by £2.75 million.There was also evidence of an improvement in social capital within the communities involved in the reducing falls programme, with improvements in the proportion of people saying the area was a good place to live and an increase in the number of people saying they felt able to make improvements in their communities.

Summary

Engaging organized groups and communities in planning and scrutiny of local health services may help to improve health outcomes. It is also the best way to ensure that health services are fit for purpose. NHS organizations have a duty to involve laypeople in governance, to ensure transparency of decision-making and to be accountable to citizens. Systems for governance and accountability must be transparent and accessible to local people. Voluntary patient organizations have much to contribute but they usually represent sectional interests only. Statutory patient groups have been established to represent the views of local patients and citizens but they have struggled to make an impact, largely because successive governments have been ambivalent about their role. Both statutory and voluntary groups can help to determine commissioning priorities, but commissioners may also need to consult with a wider range of stakeholders. Various tools and techniques are available to assist with their key tasks of assessing needs, determining priorities, service development and health promotion, all of which can benefit from community engagement.

References

Abelson, J., Eyles, J., McLeod, C.B., Collins, P., McMullan, C. and Forest, P.G. (2003) Does deliberation make a difference? Results from a citizens panel study of health goals priority setting, *Health Policy*, 66(1): 95–106.

Arnstein, S. (1969) A ladder of citizen participation, *Journal of the American Institute of Planners*, 35(4): 216–24.

Audit Commission (2003) *Corporate Governance: Improvement and Trust in Local Public Services*. London: Audit Commission.

Baggott, R., Allsop, J. and Jones, K. (2005) *Speaking for Patients and Carers: Health Consumer Groups and the Policy Process*. Basingstoke: Palgrave Macmillan.

Blackman, T., Wistow, G. and Wistow, J. (2008) *Accountability for Health: A Scoping Paper for the LGA Health Commission*. London: Local Government Association.

Boston Women's Health Book Collective (1998) *Our Bodies, Ourselves*. New York: Simon and Schuster.

Bostridge, M. (2008) *Florence Nightingale: The Woman and Her Legend*. London: Viking.

Boyle, D., Coote, A., Sherwood, C. and Slay, J. (2010) *Right Here, Right Now: Taking Co-production into the Mainstream*. London: NESTA.

Cadbury Report (1992) *The Financial Aspects of Corporate Governance*. London: Gee & Co.

Callaghan, G. and Duggan, S. (2008) Report on the evaluation of the Connected Care Audit. Durham, School of Applied Social Sciences, Durham University.

Centre for Public Scrutiny (2007) *The Anatomy of Accountability: How the National Health Service Answers to the People*. London: Centre for Public Scrutiny.

Daniels, N. and Sabin, J. (1998) The ethics of accountability in managed care reform, *Health Affairs*, 17(5): 50–64.

Department of Health (2007) *World Class Commissioning Competencies*. London: Department of Health.

Department of Health (2008) *Real Involvement: Working with People to Improve Health Services*. Available online at www.dh.gov.uk.

Department of Health (2009) *The NHS Constitution*. London: Department of Health.

Developing Patient Partnerships (NANAfPP) (2006) *Effective Practice-based Commissioning: Engaging with Local People*. London: DPP.

Dixon, S. and Shackley, P. (2003) The use of willingness to pay to assess public preferences towards the fortification of foodstuffs with folic acid, *Health Expectations*, 6(2): 140–48.

Ehrenreich, B. and English, D. (2010) *Witches, Midwives and Nurses: a History of Women Healers*, 2nd edn. New York: Feminist Press.

Goffman, E. (1961) *Asylums: Essays on the Social Situation of Mental Patients and Other Inmates*. New York: Anchor Books.

Health Development Agency (2004a) *Lessons from Health Action Zones*. London: HDA Briefing no. 9 edn. Health Development Agency.

Health Development Agency (2004b) *Social Capital for Health: Issues of Definition, Measurement and Links to Health*. London: Health Development Agency.

Healthcare Commission (2005) *Survey of Primary Care Trust Patients*. London: Commission for Healthcare Audit and Inspection.

Hogg, C. (2009) *Citizens, Consumers and the NHS: Capturing Voices*. Basingstoke: Palgrave Macmillan.

Illich, I. (1974) *Medical Nemesis*. London: Calder and Boyars.

Improvement and Development Agency (2010) *A Glass Half Full: How an Asset Approach can Improve Community Health and Wellbeing*. London: IDeA.

InHealth Associates (2009) *The Engagement Cycle: A New Way of Thinking About Patient and Public Engagement in World Class Commissioning*. Available online at www.dh.gov.uk/en/Publicationsandstatistics/Publications/PublicationsPolicyAndGuidance/DH_098658.

Involve (2010) *Public Participation Methods*. Available online at www.peopleandparticipation.net/display/Methods/Home.

Involve and togetherwecan (2005) *People and Participation*. London: Involve.

Kai, J. and Hedges, C. (1999) Minority ethnic community participation in needs assessment and service development in primary care: perceptions of Pakistani and Bangladeshi people about psychological distress, *Health Expectations*, 2(1): 7–20.

Kent, A. (2007) Should patient groups accept money from drug companies? Yes, *British Medical Journal*, 334(7600): 934.

Klein, R. (2001) *The New Politics of the NHS*. Harlow: Prentice Hall.

Kramer, R. (2010) Power to the people, *Health Service Journal*, 18 November. Available online at www.hsj.co.uk

Liverpool Primary Care Trust (2007) *The Big Health Debate*. Liverpool: Liverpool PCT.

Local Government Association Health Commission (2008) *Who's Accountable for Health? LGA Health Commission Final Report*. London: LGA.

Marmot, M. (2009) *Tackling Health Inequalities: 10 Years On*. London: Department of Health.

McKeown, T. (1976) *The Role of Medicine: Dream, Mirage or Nemesis?* London: Nuffield Provincial Hospitals Trust.

Mintzes, B. (2007) Should patient groups accept money from drug companies? No, *British Medical Journal*, 334(7600): 935.

Morgan, M.A. and Lifshay, J. (2006) *Community Engagement in Public Health*. Martinez, CA: Contra Costa Health Services.

Mullen, P.M. (1999) Public involvement in health care priority setting: an overview of methods for eliciting values, *Health Expectations*, 2(4): 222–34.

National Institute for Clinical Excellence (NICE) (2008) *Community Engagement to Improve Health*. London: NICE.

National Institute for Clinical Excellence (NICE) (2009) *Health Needs Assessment: A Practical Guide*. London: NICE.

National Leadership Centre Board Development (2010) *The Healthy NHS Board: Principles for Good Governance*. London: National Leadership Centre.

Oxford University Press (2007) *Shorter Oxford English Dictionary*. Oxford: Oxford University Press.

Picker Institute Europe (2009) *Patient and Public Engagement – The early impact of World Class Commissioning: A Survey of Primary Care Trusts*. Oxford: Picker Institute Europe.

Porter, R. (2003) *Blood and Guts: A Short History of Medicine*. London: Penguin Books.

Puska, P. (2008) The North Karelia Project: 30 Years Successfully Preventing Chronic Diseases, *Diabetes Voice*, 53: 26–29.

Putnam, R.D. (2000) *Bowling Alone: The Collapse and Revival of American community*. New York: Simon and Schuster.

Robert, G. (2003) The United Kingdom, in C. Ham and G. Robert (eds) *Reasonable Rationing* (pp. 64–93). Maidenhead: Open University Press.

Secretary of State for Health (2010) *Equity and Excellence: Liberating the NHS* (Cmd. 7881). London: The Stationery Office.

Shaw, G.B. (1906) *The Doctor's Dilemma*. London: Penguin.

Skidmore, P., Bound, K. and Lownsbrough, H. (2006) *Community Participation: Who Benefits?* York: Joseph Rowntree Foundation.

Slater, B., Knowles, J. and Lyon, D. (2008) Improvement science meets community development: approaching health inequalities through community engagement, *Journal of Integrated Care*, 16(6): 26–36.

Smith, K.E., Bambra, C., Joyce, K.E., Perkins, N., Hunter, D.J. and Blenkinsopp, E.A. (2009) Partners in health? A systematic review of the impact of organizational partnerships on public health outcomes in England between 1997 and 2008, *Journal of Public Health (Oxf)*, 31(2): 210–21.

Tudor Hart, J. (2010) *The Political Economy of Health Care*, 2nd edn. Bristol: Policy Press.

Turning Point (2010) *Connected Care*. London: Turning Point.

Weale, A. (2006) What is so good about citizens' involvement in healthcare?, in E. Andersson, J. Tritter and R. Wilson (eds) *Healthy Democracy: The Future of Involvement in Health and Social Care* (pp. 37–43). London: Involve and National Centre for Involvement.

Wood, B. (2000) *Patient Power? The Politics of Patients' Associations in Britain and America*. Maidenhead: Open University Press.

Further reading

Andersson, E., Tritter, J. and Wilson, R. (eds) (2006) *Healthy Democracy: The Future of Involvement in Health and Social Care*. London: Involve and National Centre for Involvement.

Baggott, R., Allsop, J. and Jones, K. (2005) *Speaking for Patients and Carers: Health Consumer Groups and the Policy Process*. Basingstoke: Palgrave Macmillan.

Chambers, R., Drinkwater, C. and Boath, E. (2003) *Involving Patients and the Public: How to Do It Better*, 2nd edn. Abingdon: Radcliffe Medical Press.

Davies, C., Wetherell, M. and Barnett, E. (2006) *Citizens at the Centre: Deliberative Participation in Healthcare Decisions*. Bristol: Policy Press.

Hogg C. (2009) *Citizens, Consumers and the NHS: Capturing Voices*. Basingstoke: Palgrave Macmillan.

Tudor Hart, J. (2010) *The Political Economy of Health Care*, 2nd edn. Bristol: The Policy Press.

Williamson, C. (2010) *Towards the Emancipation of Patients: Patients' Experiences and the Patient Movement*. Bristol: The Policy Press.

Wood, B. (2000) *Patient Power? The Politics of Patients' Associations in Britain and America*. Maidenhead: Open University Press.

10 Patients – the greatest untapped resource?

Overview

This chapter summarizes the conclusions of the previous chapters and considers what needs to be done to encourage greater patient and public engagement.

Assembling a balance sheet

Previous chapters in this book have suggested that patients are an untapped resource in healthcare who, if fully engaged and mobilized, could transform the quality and sustainability of health systems. The argument rests on an assertion that their potential is currently underexploited due to overdependence on technical solutions to health needs and a failure to recognize and support patients' role as key decision-makers and co-producers of health. This final chapter assembles a balance sheet to assess the extent to which this assertion is warranted.

In Chapter 1 it was suggested that patients and citizens could make an important contribution to maximizing health in at least eight distinct policy areas:

1 improving care processes
2 building health literacy
3 selecting treatments
4 strengthening self-care
5 ensuring safer care
6 participating in research
7 training professionals
8 shaping services.

What have we learnt about patients' potential and actual contribution to each of these policy priorities?

Improving care processes

While most patients give positive reports of their healthcare, there is undoubtedly potential for improvement. For a minority the experience of hospitalization can be dispiriting, disrespectful and unsafe, and care outside hospital is not always delivered as conveniently and effectively as it might be. The NHS has invested heavily in measuring patients' experience since the first national patient surveys were launched in England in 2002, but this type of feedback has not yet proved sufficiently powerful to drive up quality without additional stimuli. Health professionals and provider organizations will require stronger incentives to take note of the results of patient surveys or patients' stories and take appropriate action. This area has lacked effective clinical and managerial leadership to date.

Whether the increased emphasis on competition and choice will prove to be an effective remedy remains to be seen. It might do so, especially if the availability and presentation of performance information improves, but evidence in support of this policy is not strong as yet. In the meantime, emphasizing patients' rights to receive care that meets certain quality standards and encouraging the public to expect high-quality care and push for it may be more effective. Certainly the success of the waiting times initiative has demonstrated that targets backed up by central directives can be effective.

Centrally driven initiatives to raise quality standards will not succeed unless they are matched by effective action from staff on the ground. Changing entrenched organizational processes is often difficult. Some healthcare organizations have found that directly involving patients in describing their experiences and suggesting improvements can be very helpful. While there is much enthusiasm for this approach, more research is needed to evaluate the precise effects of patient participation on the quality and effectiveness of services.

Building health literacy

The public has a huge thirst for information about health and healthcare. Health professionals have a responsibility to educate and inform patients and to boost their confidence and skills for making decisions about their health. Often this means a radical change in how medical consultations are conducted, with less emphasis on giving instructions and advice, and more on encouraging patients to determine their own goals and helping them to meet them. Information can have a therapeutic role, improving people's ability to cope with illness and enhancing their ability to look after themselves, so clinicians should help patients to access it.

The Internet has transformed people's ability to find relevant information. Assessing the reliability of this information is difficult however, and much of it is of poor quality. The popular media can play an important role in increasing understanding of health issues, but many media stories are biased and unreliable. There is limited evidence of effective use of educational techniques to reduce the health gap between rich and poor, but specially designed initiatives targeted at disadvantaged groups can lead to significant improvements in people's knowledge and coping ability. Enabling people to make sense of what they read and hear about health and healthcare and critically assess it should be a central plank of any public health strategy.

Selecting treatments

Patients' preferences should guide treatment decision-making, with patients being helped to select treatments that produce the best match with their values, outcome preferences and tolerance of risk. This involves making sure that patients have access to reliable, evidence-based information about the treatment options and likely outcomes, and guiding them through a deliberation process designed to identify the best option for them. Many patients want this level of involvement, but clinicians often fail to inform and engage them, despite an ethical commitment to informed consent. Patient decision aids provide accurate, comprehensible information and decision support and they have proved to be both acceptable and useful, but they have been slow to filter into the mainstream of clinical practice.

Many people, clinicians as well as patients, struggle to understand and interpret data on probabilities. The problem is often exacerbated by the confusing way in which research findings are communicated in medical journals; for example, reporting results in terms of relative risk rather than absolute risk. This can leave readers believing that treatment effects are greater than they really are. Understanding could be greatly improved if researchers, journal editors, clinicians and journalists were to follow guidelines for clear communication of risk. The goal is to improve decision quality, ensuring that patients receive only the tests and procedures they want and need, no more and no less. Despite considerable enthusiasm for this approach and a relatively robust evidence base, shared decision-making is not yet the norm in mainstream clinical practice.

Strengthening self-care

People with chronic disease have to deal with the effects of their long-term conditions. They must administer their own treatment, often on a daily basis, monitor their symptoms, and learn how to avoid future exacerbations by adopting healthy lifestyles. Many patients with these conditions do not currently receive sufficient support from health professionals to self-manage effectively. Despite numerous policy commitments to the promotion of a collaborative approach, implementation remains a challenge.

Self-management education is one response to the problem that has been tried quite extensively. Whether patient-led programmes are as effective as professionally led ones is much disputed, but the social support they provide is usually welcomed by participants. The goal is to strengthen and maintain people's independence, reducing the need for medical consultation or hospitalization and enabling people with multiple health problems to remain in their own homes for as long as possible. Collaborative care planning should be the norm for long-term conditions, but staff need training in how to do this effectively. Health coaching and web-based support can be helpful, as can other remote technologies such as movement sensors, telemonitors and automated reminders. Giving patients access to their medical records and encouraging them to review them appears to offer benefits, but few people in the UK have had this opportunity as yet, and many GPs appear reluctant to encourage it. Similarly, the ability to consult doctors by email has been slower to develop in the UK than in some other countries.

Evidence shows that it is possible to significantly increase people's knowledge and understanding of their condition, but information alone has little impact on symptoms or behaviours. Some approaches have led to positive short-term effects on people's confidence and coping ability, but few studies have looked at whether these skills are sustained in the longer term. Studies of the impact of self-management support on health behaviour and health status have produced mixed results, with different outcomes for different conditions. Published studies of cost-effectiveness are relatively rare, but a small number have indicated that effective support for self-management might help to reduce healthcare costs.

Ensuring safer care

Patients can be victims of medical mistakes, but they can also be part of the safety solution. Among several suggestions for improving safety in hospitals, there has been considerable interest in building awareness of issues such as hospital-acquired infections or survival following surgery, by publishing the rates on public websites. The intention is to bring pressure to bear on those institutions with poor safety records, because referring clinicians and patients will avoid them, hopefully sending signals that will stimulate greater efforts to improve. But as yet it has not been proven that publishing performance data improves safety and most patients and GPs do not make use of this information when choosing providers. Whether the problem lies in the way the data are presented (which could of course be improved), or whether it is more fundamental (perhaps related to the way people make decisions in the real world), must await the results of more and better studies. Encouraging greater public awareness of safety issues makes sense, as does emphasizing the need for honesty, transparency and apologies when things go wrong.

Poor quality communication and the mistakes that arise from this are a major cause of error in diagnosis. Patient-centred consulting styles, in which the doctor takes time to elicit and listen to the patient's description of their symptoms, concerns and medical history, increase the likelihood that important information will be shared, hence reducing the risk of error. Efforts to ensure that patients are kept fully informed about their medicines, including what they are, how they are supposed to work, the reasons for prescribing them, the correct dosage, how to take them, and any likely side-effects, are essential. Strange as it may seem, patients are often not provided with this information in a way that they can understand and readily implement.

Participating in research

Patients have been involved in helping to identify research priorities since the launch of the NHS research and development programme in 1991. However, there is often a mismatch between what gets funded and what patients consider important and the research agenda is still largely shaped by commercial interests and regulatory requirements.

Patients are often more interested in knowing about the likely impact of treatments on their physical and emotional functioning than on biomedical indicators. The use of patient reported outcome measures (PROMs) increases the likelihood that studies will investigate topics of relevance to patients, offering greater potential to inform their treatment choices. To achieve this, the results must be made available in an accessible and comprehensible form, readily accessible when needed. However, there are few incentives for researchers to devote time to producing summaries of their findings for use by patients and members of the public.

Training professionals

Professional regulators expect doctors, nurses and allied health professionals to reach competent standards in communicating with patients, sharing decisions and supporting self-care. Detailed curricula have been developed incorporating these topics, and it is clear that the relevant skills can be taught. But trainees enter a clinical world that places greater value on technical competences than on interpersonal skills, and the hidden curriculum often swamps what they have learnt during their formal training.

Involving patients directly as teachers, using actors as simulated patients, organizing mixed professional groups to learn together, and providing opportunities for community-based learning, are promising developments, but research into the effects of these various approaches is in its infancy and there is little hard evidence available to guide patient-centred curriculum planning and course design.

Shaping services

Achieving wider engagement in determining health needs, and ensuring that services are fit for purpose, means allowing all relevant stakeholders to have their say. Voluntary patient organizations have an important role to play, but too often their efforts have been fragmented and coordination has proved problematic. Meanwhile the statutory patient groups have had a chequered history, and their impact has been weakened by frequent shifts in government policy and several reorganizations.

A variety of methods have been developed to assist commissioners in the process of engaging with local people. Some have used these to good effect, while others have found the task too challenging. While engaging with local communities seems self-evidently worth while, determining the best way to go about it and measuring its impact requires more careful evaluation than it has received to date.

Strengthening impact

So is it true that patients are an untapped resource? Not entirely, since we have reviewed several examples where they have been engaged as active participants, often with good results. There have also been numerous policy initiatives designed to strengthen their role, as we have seen. But many of the practical examples were isolated demonstration projects and many of the policies failed to translate rhetoric into practical action. Fully informed and engaged patients are by no means the norm and mainstream clinical practice remains resistant to these developments.

The evidence reviewed in this book suggests there is considerable potential to improve effectiveness and efficiency in healthcare if only patients were more actively engaged. For patients to play an active role in their own healthcare and that of their communities, they must be better supported, better informed, encouraged to be more discriminating about the effects of medical treatment, and have more opportunities for participation. What more can be done to encourage this?

Personalizing care

Most people want to look after their own and their family's health as best they can, but they often need more effective support from health professionals to do so. Supporting self-care and self-management should be given much greater priority in professional training programmes and these skills should be assessed. Patients should have a choice of care packages whenever appropriate and care plans should be personalized to their specific needs and circumstances. They should be given access to evidence-based clinical guidelines to inform them about what ought to happen during a care pathway so they can check that they have received recommended treatment and monitoring. Self-management education programmes should be made more widely available, tailored to the needs of particular groups. Help with making lifestyle changes should be available for those who want it, supported by health coaches trained in motivational interviewing, and by web-based packages or peer support groups. All patients should have the opportunity to book appointments and order repeat prescriptions online, a facility that is available to only a small minority at present. Different healthcare services should be integrated where possible and well coordinated to ensure continuity of care, and there should be special help for those with multiple needs to remain independent for as long as possible.

Prioritizing health literacy

There is already a great deal of health information available for those who seek it out, but it should be delivered more proactively so that it is always available when people need it to inform their decisions. Policy-makers should prioritize health literacy and commit to raising standards by various means, including formal and informal education, information provision and better communication. Health professionals should capitalize on opportunities to educate patients and they should signpost information more effectively, offering information prescriptions alongside medications and other treatments.

Electronic medical records, including copies of referral letters and test results, should always be accessible to patients as well as professionals, with embedded links to information and support at relevant decision points. Websites and printed information should be evaluated and certified to show they meet agreed quality standards. Patient decision aids should be made available covering all common conditions, diagnostic tests and treatments, linked into medical records and delivered electronically. People should be able to use interactive websites, email or call centres to consult health professionals about specific health problems and to give and receive feedback on the quality of services. Mobile phones and other wireless applications could help to make health information accessible to a wider audience, capitalizing on the interest in social networking to provide virtual support to promote health. Wherever possible, health information should be tailored to those with special needs and made available on appropriate media.

Demystifying medical knowledge

Producers and providers of medical treatments and services are expert at generating demand for their products. They do this by publicizing the benefits, downplaying the risks and encouraging dependency on their knowledge and expertise. Countering this tendency involves demystifying expert know-how by presenting it in terms that ordinary people can understand, encouraging patients to ask questions and be more discriminating, and boosting their confidence to make their own decisions. Clinicians should be given incentives to ensure that patients are fully informed about treatment options and supported to make healthcare choices. They should be trained to communicate risk more effectively and to share decisions and treatment plans, supported by appropriate tools and techniques. Their performance in respect of shared decision-making and collaborative care planning should be monitored and good practice rewarded. Medical journals could do a better job of reporting outcome probabilities in terms that are readily comprehensible to clinicians and journalists. The quality of health journalism could be improved by providing training, publicizing editorial guidelines, and reporting abuses.

Engaging citizens

NHS organizations already have a duty to involve patients in evaluating services and they must consult local people before making changes. All citizens have an interest in ensuring that healthcare resources are expended effectively, efficiently and equitably, so their views on priorities should be listened to. Greater effort could be made to keep people informed about practice variations, quality problems, and resource allocation dilemmas, with a view to fostering more informed debate about health policy issues.

A high-quality health service is one that is both organized around, and responsive to, the needs of the people who use it. Recognizing and strengthening the patient's role may be the best hope there is for ensuring that healthcare remains effective and affordable into the future.

Index

Locators shown in *italics* refer to figures and tables.

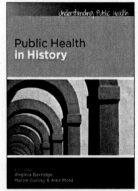

PUBLIC HISTORY AND HEALTH

Virginia Berridge, Martin Gorsky and Alex Mold

9780335242641 (Paperback)
2011

eBook also available

This book offers unique introduction to key themes in the history of medicine, health and public health and is designed as reading for a range of healthcare students.

The book combines wide ranging history of medicine with a contemporary look at public health issues, and is a fascinating overview of the history of 'health'. Looking at health developments in the 19th and 20th centuries in a range of different countries and contexts, the book includes case studies on malaria, smallpox and more modern health issues challenges such as AIDS and substance abuse

This is the definitive history of public health designed to engage and excite a wide range of health professionals.

Key features:

- Interactive exercises for students based on primary source material
- Includes major case study chapters, covering developments in medicine and public health history
- Written by experts from the London School of Tropical Medicine

www.openup.co.uk

OPEN UNIVERSITY PRESS
McGraw - Hill Education

Understanding
Health
Inequalities

SECOND EDITION

Edited by HILARY GRAHAM

UNDERSTANDING HEALTH INEQUALITIES 2/E

Hilary Graham

9780335234592 (Paperback)
2009

eBook also available

Understanding Health Inequalities second edition provides an accessible and engaging exploration of why the opportunity to live a long and healthy life remains profoundly unequal.

Hilary Graham and her contributors outline the enduring link between people's socioeconomic circumstances and their health and tackle questions at the forefront of research and policy on health inequalities. These include:

- How health is influenced by circumstances across people's lives and by the areas in which they live
- How health is simultaneously shaped by inequalities of gender, ethnicity and socioeconomic position
- How policies can impact on health inequalities

All the chapters have been specially written for the new edition by internationally-recognised researchers in social and health inequalities. The book provides an authoritative guide to these fields as well as presenting new research.

www.openup.co.uk

OPEN UNIVERSITY PRESS
McGraw - Hill Education

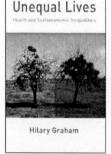

UNEQUAL LIVES: HEALTH AND SOCIOECONOMIC INEQUALITIES

Hilary Graham

0335213693 (Paperback)
2009

eBook also available

"With the compelling evidence that more redistributive universal welfare benefits and education provide the main escalator to reducing inequalities, this is a timely and thought-provoking book for all those concerned to reduce our societies' embedded structural inequalities, cumulative disadvantages and health inequalities."
Australian and New Zealand Journal of Public Health.

- What is meant by health inequalities and socioeconomic inequalities?
- What evidence is there to support the link between socioeconomic status and health?
- Why do these links persist over time, between and within societies, and across people's lives?
- What part do policies play in the persistence of social and health inequalities?

Unequal Lives provides an evidence-based introduction to social and health inequalities. It brings together research from social epidemiology, sociology and social policy to guide the reader to an understanding of why people's lives and people's health remain so unequal, even in rich societies where there is more than enough for all.

www.openup.co.uk

OPEN UNIVERSITY PRESS
McGraw - Hill Education

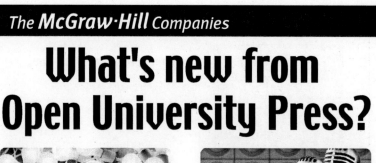
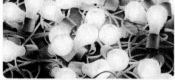
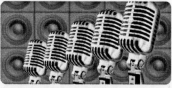
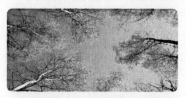
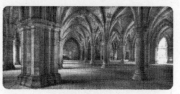
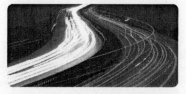
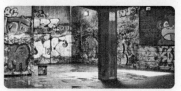

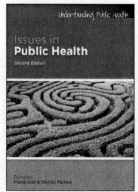

PUBLIC HISTORY AND HEALTH 2/E

Fiona Sim and Martin McKee

9780335242641 (Paperback)
2011

eBook also available

Issues in Public Health, second edition is a text for those who want to answer the questions, 'What is public health?' and 'Why is it important?'.

This book looks at the foundations of public health, its historical evolution, the themes that underpin public health, the increasing importance of globalization and the most important causes of avoidable disease and injury. These include:

- Environmental factors
- Tobacco
- Nutrition
- Personal lifestyle factors
- Infectious disease

The second edition includes new chapters on the expanding role of public health and the impact of climate change on health. It also features expanded examples of the impact of globalization on higher and lower income countries and explores the tension between the population approach and the personal behaviour change model of health promotion.

www.openup.co.uk

OPEN UNIVERSITY PRESS
McGraw · Hill Education

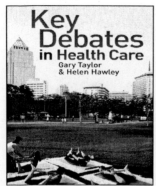

KEY DEBATES IN HEALTHCARE

Gary Taylor and Helen Hawley

9780335223947 (Paperback)
2010

eBook also available

The book examines the different models of health and healthcare delivery, and explores alternative methods of providing healthcare, using the state, the private sector or the voluntary sector. Through these debates the book will help readers explore issues such as health inequalities, health promotion and service delivery, and establish their own perspective on issues of health and society.

Key features:

- Theoretical perspectives to help understand the logic and implications of broad social and political arguments related to health
- Policy developments to show the practical application of ideas in Britain, the United States and in other parts of the world
- Healthcare scenarios to help make connections between theory, policy and practice

www.openup.co.uk

OPEN UNIVERSITY PRESS
McGraw - Hill Education

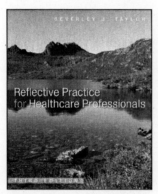

**REFLECTIVE PRACTICE FOR
HEALTHCARE PROFESSIONALS**
Third Edition

Beverley J. Taylor

9780335238354 (Paperback)
2010

eBook also available

This popular book provides practical guidance for healthcare professionals
wishing to reflect on their work and improve the way they undertake clinical
procedures, interact with other people at work and deal with power issues. The
new edition has been broadened in focus from nurses and midwives exclusively,
to include all healthcare professionals.

Key features:

- Identifies the fundamentals of reflective practice and how and why it is
  embraced in healthcare professions
- Includes strategies for effective reflection
- Provides a step-by-step guide to applying the Taylor REFLECT model

www.openup.co.uk

OPEN UNIVERSITY PRESS
McGraw · Hill Education